There are flowers in the desert

by

Audrey Aspeling

The true story of a nursing experience in outback Australia

1971–1974

Audrey Aspeling.

23 Dublin Road
Ringwood East
Vic. 3135, Australia
Tel: (03) 9870 2213

Seaview Press
PO Box 234
Henley Beach, South Australia 5022
Telephone 08 8235 1535; fax 08 8235 9144
E-mail: seaview@seaviewpress.com.au
Web site: http://www.seaviewpress.com.au

Printed by:
Copy Master
234 Currie Street
Adelaide, South Australia 5000

Cover design: John Low-Shang.
Cover photo: Audrey Aspeling. "The flowers of the desert."
Author's photo 1999: Negley Aspeling.
Author's photo 1971 taken just before going to Laverton W.A.: Hedley Candids Photographers, Kalgoorlie. W.A.

National Library of Australia Cataloguing-in-Publication entry
Aspeling, Audrey.
There are flowers in the desert : the true story of a nursing experience in outback Australia 1971-1974.

ISBN 1 74008 088 2.

1. Aspeling, Audrey. 2. Bush Church Aid Society (Australia).
3. Nurses - Australia - Biography. I. Title.

610.73092

Dedicated to The Bush Church Aid Society of Australia,
and to all those who over past years have willingly
left the security of their homes to venture
into the more remote areas of our
country to assist the people there.
Theirs has been an oft
unsung, but no
less valuable
contribution.

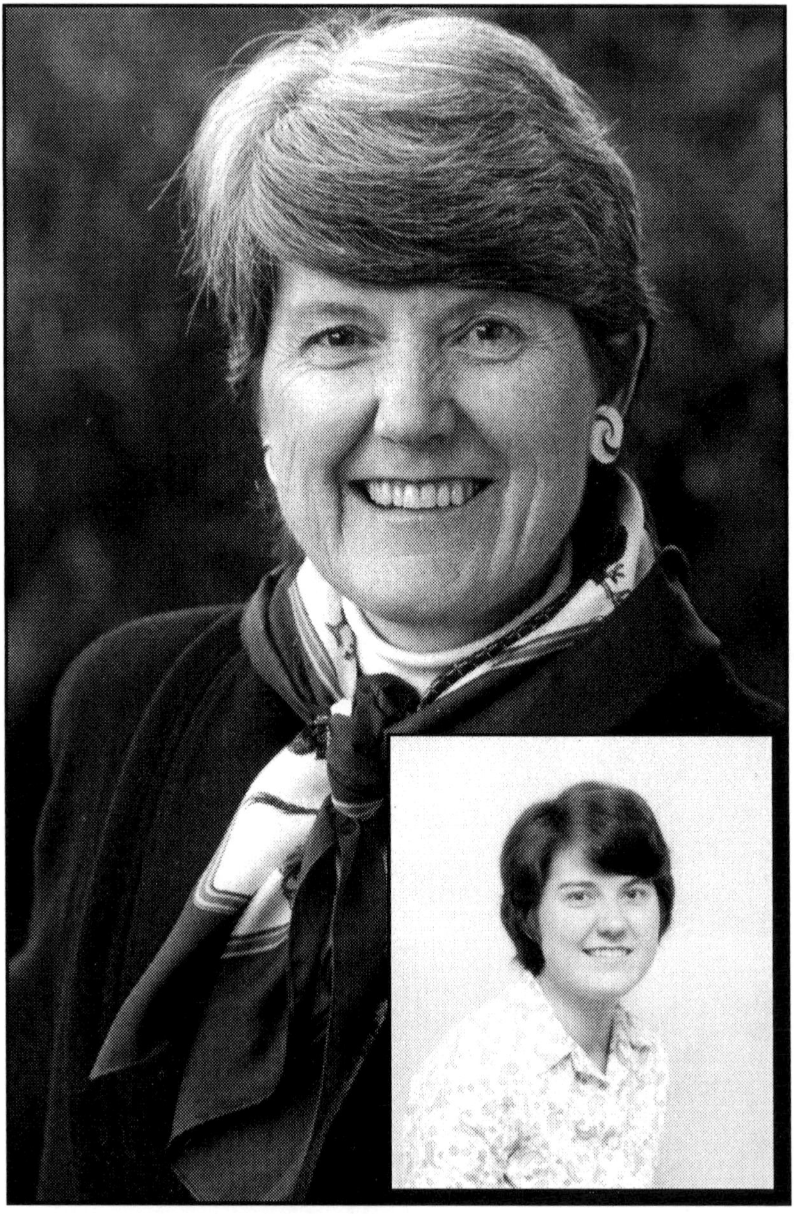

Audrey Aspeling in 1999 (Photo: Negley Aspeling);
inset in 1971

ABOUT THE AUTHOR

Audrey Aspeling was born Audrey Nixon on the 13th of December 1945, the second daughter of an Anglican Clergyman in country Victoria, Australia. She was brought up as a church going Anglican whose mother suffered a complete physical and mental breakdown when Audrey was 8 years old. At the age of 11, Audrey took herself out of the home environment, and into an Anglican boarding school (Queens in Ballarat) which she thoroughly enjoyed for 5 years. Her academic ability was very adequate, but she had practically no ambition and absolutely no idea of what she wanted to do with her life. Her mother recovered and tried to instil some ambition into this daughter, and finally Audrey decided to become a nurse, mostly because of the uniform, the sensible shoes, and she couldn't think of anything else! After the first eight classroom weeks of Preliminary Training School, marked by her perception of expected traumas in this job, Audrey met up with bedside nursing and never looked back.

After completing the basic course and a Staff Nurse year at the Royal Melbourne Hospital in 1967, Audrey undertook obstetrics at Crown Street Women's Hospital in Sydney. It was there where she first met Jesus in a personal way and decided to accept Him as her Lord and Saviour. An earlier contact with the Bush Church Aid Society (B.C.A.) of Australia came back to her with new meaning, and after more obstetric experience and the completion of a Maternal and Child Health course, Audrey went out as a nurse with B.C.A. in March 1971.

ACKNOWLEDGEMENTS

Firstly my heartfelt thanks must go to my Mum and Dad, Mary and Eric Nixon, who, I believe, set my childhood feet firmly on the right path when they taught me from the very beginning to have faith in God. Unfortunately they are not alive to share in the completion of this book. Secondly, my thanks to my husband Negley, my sister Tricia, my mother-in-law Bessie and my father-in-law Ivan (Ivan is also now deceased), for their long-term unfailing support throughout the protracted and sometimes arduous preparation of the book. Without them I may never have reached the end of the project. Thirdly to Carol, my B.C.A. friend and colleague, my gratitude for always believing in the value of the work.

I would also like to thank most sincerely the members of the Bush Church Aid Society family who have read and accepted the book, and are still supporting it with their advice and promotional ideas, and to Barry Green for his foreword.

Special thanks to John and Lorraine Low-Shang, friends and helpers when the going got tough, Graham at Hot Pepper Studios in Ringwood, Renee at Smith's Photos and Matt at Bond Colour, for helping me organise my slides for inclusion, and to all my work colleagues, relatives, and friends, especially my near neighbours Gladys, Rebecca, Grace, Ann, Una, and Bonnie, who have not only taken interest, but have listened seemingly tirelessly to my endless discourses on the subject.

Finally and most importantly of all, none of this would have happened or been able to be written about, if it were not for God, His Son Jesus Christ, and the leading of His Holy Spirit in my life. The experience of this has been the ultimate fulfilment.

FOREWORD

To most Christians in Australia their faith is lived out in a community of 'fellow believers'. New Christians have the safeguard of being nurtured by other more experienced folk. There is the choice of congregations and different age mixes, ethnic groups and denominational groups as well as the joy of meeting together at joint occasions where one simply accepts the fact that there will be talented musicians and speakers and exciting facilities.

When a person is removed from these facilities and choices, and finds oneself living in an isolated community with little choice…no regular worship facilities or musicians, and no 'leader'…the goal posts are moved and the situation changes. The person—whether new to the Faith or experienced—finds himself/herself having to learn a new way to live out that Faith!

In many areas covered by the ministry of The Bush Church Aid Society, this is the case.

Audrey's book gives an honest and from the heart look at such a transition, and gives us a rare chance to examine our own responses through her experiences.

The Revd. Barry W. Green
Ex. B.C.A. Missioner and State Secretary.

INTRODUCTION

This book, in an autobiographical genre, shares the threads of circumstance which led to the author's sojourn in three different areas of central Australia, over a three-year period. It chronicles her fears, failures, and God-given successes in the outback, seeking Australia for Christ as a nurse with the Bush Church Aid Society. It includes stories of the spiritual and the nursing work, romance, and culture, and describes each area visited with images of the type of terrain, the lifestyle, the weather, and the people who lived there. The discussion about Aboriginal Australians leads to the discovery of some of their problems as well as their charms, plus the relative relationships between black and white which vary according to the different areas visited.

The vastness and isolation of the Australian desert comes through, along with the essence of loneliness, which is at times crushing. Good relationships are crucial, and yet difficult to find. The normal props we all take for granted in city life are totally absent in some parts, and strategies for dealing with this are described. In all this emptiness it is discovered that if one is open to learn from the experience, one can eventually find oneself really loving the uniqueness of the task and basking in its differences.

Through her writings the author hopes that not only will the reader be convinced that "There ARE Flowers in the Desert", but that the spirit of God might also flower in the life of each person who takes the time to read these pages.

HISTORICAL FACTS OF THE EARLY 1970s

Notes from the Author

LAVERTON, W.A.

Laverton was originally a gold-mining town, which boomed from 1898 and was gazetted as a town on July 6 1900. The mining prospered up until World War 1 when the men left for the war effort, and again in the 1930s, until the commencement of World War 2. After the gold rush subsided, growth in the area did not recover until Western Mining commenced nickel mining in 1968. Nickel transformed Laverton, and in 1975, when the population grew again, the mining company completely rebuilt the town.

At the time referred to in the book, Laverton's Aboriginals were members of the Wongi tribe, most of whom lived on a reserve on the town's outer edge, near to the Laverton Government Hospital. The nickel boom developed just after the experiences outlined, so the picture at the time of writing, was of a small remnant of whites from the gold days, a new beginning influx of white mining company workers investigating the possibilities of future nickel successes, and a fringe of black Australians living in a kind of separated tolerance, where black and white had little to do with each other. Though based at the reserve, many Aboriginals in Laverton still hunted kangaroo, built their campfires, and went walkabout. Complete integration of the white and black cultures looked to be a long way off.

COOK S.A.

Cook was a railway town born expressly for the purpose of servicing the trains travelling across the Nullarbor Plain, and maintaining the railway tracks. This small settlement appeared to exhibit true harmony between black and white inhabitants. All lived in the same type of houses, did the same sorts of jobs (that is working for the Commonwealth of Australia Railways), and maintained similar lifestyles. Here seemed to be true integration, but unfortunately this came at the price of the complete loss of Aboriginal culture.

COOBER PEDY S.A.

Coober Pedy was a booming opal-mining town, rough, dusty, and vibrant with successes, failures, and dreams. White men mined via drill holes and open cuts, while local Aboriginals and others noodled (meaning they sat on the piles of drilled out dust, and sifted out the opal remnants thrown to one side by the miners' methods). Most of the Aboriginals here had also lost their culture totally, but were unable to replace it with anything of value for them. Some were addicted to alcohol, and most ate easily obtained refined sugar diets, instead of the healthy foods they had eaten in their original untainted lifestyle. Generally they had succumbed to the not always helpful white influences, and seemed powerless to change their situation. They were however, more integrated than those in Laverton, and one might have thought their progress towards assimilation might have had more success, if, that is, assimilation is the right choice for these displaced people, whose loss of their own rich culture, though possibly unavoidable, has been a tragedy. The passages at the end of this book show that, unfortunately up to 1998 there has not been much change for the good for Aboriginals in Coober Pedy, and for whatever reason Laverton seems to have been more successful. This could be due to the fact that Laverton is now a company town with company money assisting Government funded enterprises, whereas Coober Pedy is a group of individuals seeking their own fortunes, mostly without any company-type backing.

Through the eyes of the author, this book gives some insights into her own life before and during her bush nursing experience, the lives of some of the people described in the three places above, and the lives of those who moved into and out of their worlds from other parts of Australia and even from overseas. This is just one of the many stories which could be told of Outback Nursing, Christian Living, and the Work of the Bush Church Aid Society of Australia.

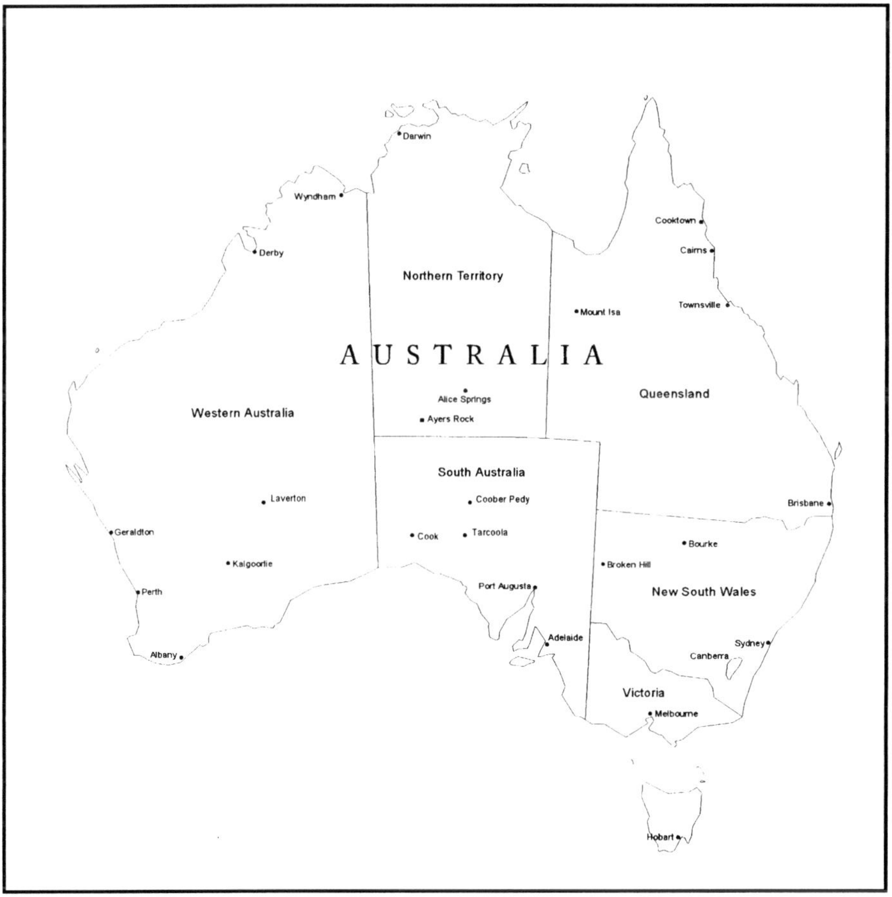

CONTENTS

CHAPTER 1 DESTINY'S FINGERTIPS

Ballarat 1958–62

The sunlight shone, its slanting rays like shafts through the small squares of glass which made up the large windows of the school hall. As usual, we were all seated on row upon row of bench type chairs, minds wandering along paths of childhood imagination while the missionary speaker's voice droned on. At 12 years of age it may be difficult to see the point of listening to missionary stories, and one might have been tempted to ignore the issue completely, but for me the impact was different. For some absolutely unknown reason I was fearful. Fearful of the fact that one day God might expect me to make a sacrifice of myself in this way. That's how I saw it, even at that tender age. This was a church boarding school I had chosen to attend and I loved. My belief was that if one were to do what God wanted with one's life one would be OK. Why then was I afraid?

Assembly over we surged out of the hall and along the corridor to our respective classrooms. The missionary theme moved out of my mind, as it filled with other things, both academic and personal. My fears dissipated and I was able to forget about it. That is until the next speaker came along, and then the same surges of emotion would relentlessly resurface.

Apart from this, for me boarding school was fun. Not everyone thought so of course, but then not everyone chose his or her own destiny as I did. My mother had been ill since I was 8 years old, and though saddened by the thought, she did not oppose my request to go away to school. I had been an avid reader of schoolgirl stories. "Real boarding schools are not like those described in books," said one of the headmistresses who interviewed me when I applied for scholarships. I didn't believe her, and luckily the school which finally took me on, was pretty much as I had hoped it would be.

There were midnight feasts. We stayed awake one hour each, creeping across the dormitory to wake the next watch at the end of our turn. Midnight would arrive and the excitement was electric, making it difficult to be as quiet as we needed to avoid detection. Pavlovas, cakes, lollies etc. smuggled in, courtesy of the day-girls' co-operation, were laid out on a cloth on the floor, and we sat around, giggling as we revelled in uncontrolled consumption of all that we loved to eat. No thought was given at the time, to the inevitable feelings of unwellness which would greet us when we awoke the next morning. It was worth it.

We actually worked hard at our studies as well. There seemed to be a competition in our class as to who could do the most! Maybe that was a legacy of an 'all girls' boarding school as opposed to co-ed. "What time are you getting up in the morning?" Robyn would ask. "Why should we tell her?" we used to think. "She only wants to do more study than us and get better marks." Amazing but true, this atmosphere of wanting to be the best in the class prevailed.

The other aspects of this school were good too. We were encouraged to play sport every day, and the meals were excellent, except for having to eat lumpy custard and lemon sago when even the thought of these things nauseated me. Every weekend we were taken on an outing of general choice. It could be to a movie, for a hike, or to one of the local special events such as Ballarat's beautiful Begonia Festival. The begonias were large colourful flowers, each petal so perfect that at times it was hard to believe that these flowers were real. Then there was the almost endless procession of decorated floats which were driven past us down the main street as we stood on the side of the road enjoying someone else's creativity. Generally not allowed out of the school grounds except for supervised events such as these, and of course to attend the weekly church service at the Anglican cathedral, we always enjoyed these outings. We even went occasionally to the drive-in theatre in a bus. My sister at home was amazed when I told her we had been to see Elvis Presley in "Jailhouse Rock"!

I used to walk across the hockey field on bright sunny days and think to myself: "I really love this place." It didn't matter to me that there were rules, regulations, and routines. That was part of what made it good, because at home from the time of my mother's illness, things had been somewhat disorganised and insecure. For me this place was an oasis.

Having lived in various small towns, courtesy of my father's occupation as an Anglican minister of religion, when I went to boarding school first, we lived in Maldon in central Victoria. Maldon was an old gold-mining town which at that time had little else besides a primary school, five hotels, two butcher shops and a shoe store. Set in the midst of hilly countryside with scenic views whichever way one chose to look, Maldon was a very pretty place, but psychologically barren. Brought up in the city, my mother hated it. The vicarage where we lived, was a place of horror to Mum, especially when the rain poured in through the vestibule windows and flooded the house. I still remember her distraught look that day when we came home from school.

It had rained heavily for some time, when suddenly the water flowed in without warning, the ensuing waterfall seemingly unstoppable. My mother stood helpless, watching the flagstone floor become the bottom of an internal mini-lake. Tears dissolved her usually stoic countenance. In sharing previous country assignments with her clergyman husband, my mother had survived two Caesarean section deliveries when giving birth to my sister and I, numerous duststorms in the dryer places, always an inadequate monetary income, and a previous abode which did not even boast of a bathroom. As well, there were always the Pharisaic-like criticisms from some of the so-called Christians of the town, which seemed to be the general lot of the country vicar's wife, and now a flood! From her point of view, it was just too much. However, despite my mother's traumas and the effects of them on our family, in my childishness, I loved Maldon.

Having a vivid imagination at that age, I revelled in the mysterious flavour of an old rambling home set in scrubby unkempt bushland in the quiet of this small Australian country town. The house was not only old and large, but also built of brick, and uniquely cut into the side of a hill. A big verandah at the front was reached via several wide stone steps, and the front door led into a long, spacious, hallway, with two very large rooms off each side, and a door at the far end. On first entry, that door could be conjured up to be the entrance to any kind of fantasy world that a small child could possibly wish to construct, and I was really into those sorts of mind games. But in reality, this door opened into the now defamed vestibule, and once in there, to the right, was yet another door, through which lay three rooms open to the outside at the back. These were reputed to have been the servants' quarters originally, and now my father used one of them for a study. Back in the vestibule and three more steps up, a small area led to the pantry and small cellar ahead, the old bathroom with chip heater to the right, and an old-style kitchen with wood-fuelled stove on the left. At that time, dishwashers, refrigerators, and built-in cupboards were unheard of. Food was bought fresh or kept in a mesh-walled cupboard called a Coolgardie safe, wet hessian around it so that the air blowing through would cool the contents. Free standing cabinets, or in my parent's poverty-stricken case, crates with a coloured curtain over the front to keep out the dust, held crockery, cutlery, and other kitchen items, while more durable foodstuffs, including home bottled everything you could think of, were stored on the pantry shelves and in the cellar. This was definitely before the days of tinned and packaged provisions.

We drank tank water, and used the town supply of tap water for everything else, but of course there was no hot water supply either. One heated the kettle on the wood stove for the dishes, and the chip heater already mentioned, in the bathroom, was lit up before a bath to heat the water.

The back door opened from the kitchen, and one was immediately confronted with the rockface, out of which the deep niche for the house had been carved. The laundry lay to the right of the back door. In those days there was no washing machine either, only a copper and tubs. The copper water was heated by a wood fire underneath, and here the washing boiled away in such a manner that any dirt, either real or imagined, could not possibly have survived. The wooden potstick was dexterously used to transfer the hot fabrics to the rinsing water in the tubs, and on to the hand-wound ringer to squeeze out the water. The glass washboard with a wooden frame around it, was used to rub the clothes against to remove any stubborn stains. From the laundry, one had to carry the washing along the back path and up more steps to the old single wire clothesline on the hilltop above. The line was held up in the air with a wooden prop which was lowered to hang things out, and raised up again for drying in the warm sunshine and hopefully a stiff breeze.

Above the clothesline area was the church hall, surrounded by bush, and built likewise of solid brick. The toilet was also outdoors at the back, along another little pathway to the right, some distance from the house. This was a pan model, emptied weekly by the night soil man. Visiting the toilet in the dark was fearful in the extreme, especially for children. A candle was always necessary, but one still dreamt of red-back spiders and tiger snakes which were prevalent in the area. The pot under the bed was definitely the best idea for middle of the night use!

My imagination which I enjoyed so much, unfortunately sometimes led to family misunderstandings. "I think you should take Audrey to a Doctor Mum, she's mad" said my sister one day. "Why on earth would you say that" my mother countered. "She's sitting up in the mulberry tree talking to herself" my sister replied. "Leave her alone" Mum instructed. "She's just exercising the fantasies of 11 years of age." I think that was how I coped with the home problems caused by my mother's unwellness, but boarding school had released me from all that. No longer did I seem to need my own private world to escape from the daily grind. The real life of school was an adventure in itself.

A lot of the other things we did at school every year also gave us pleasure. Initiation ceremonies for new pupils were particularly fascinating. The main boarding house was a gracious, old, two-story home, with a tower and a cellar. The latter was said to be a wartime retreat, which was supposed to have originally stretched underground beneath the tennis courts and the hockey field, across to the other boarding house. The former, we decided, led to other mysteries. We told our newcomers that the heart of an old headmistress was buried under the sixteenth step up to the tower! We would get a liver from the kitchen, place it in a box, blindfold the poor victim, and make them feel Miss Hayhoe's heart.

Neither the tower nor the cellar was supposed to be accessed by any of us, that being the reason for the padlocks on the doors leading to these places. We all managed to tour both however, having perfected the art of slipping the locks. Just as well nothing untoward occurred, as the areas were said to be unsafe, and the cellar had already fallen in completely just a little inside, precluding us from ever knowing if the tunnel really went as far as it was reputed to have done.

I continued at this wonderful place for five years, academically reaching and completing the year 12 certificate, listening to many missionary speakers over the time, and always feeling afraid. My only consolation with this fear was that I thought to myself, "Even if I couldn't feel comfortable with overseas missionary work, I could go to the Australian outback". What a strange thought, and why did it even enter the equation of my life at that time? I had no idea.

CHAPTER 2 SEARCHING FOR ANSWERS

Melbourne 1963–68

The word ambition was not in my vocabulary. My mother despaired of what she would do with me. I wanted in a way to become a Doctor, but felt that this was no life for a woman in the 1960s in Australia. If I was going to get married and have children eventually, what a waste of six years training and two years internship, to just leave it all when the right man came along, which I hoped would not be too far into the future. I had passed my year 12 subjects with reasonably good grades, but as the subjects taken were more attune to what I enjoyed rather than what I hoped to do with them, I had half humanities and half sciences, precluding me at that time, from specialising in either area.

"Why don't you go and do a secretarial course while you are working out what you will do eventually?" my mother suggested. I didn't disagree with this, but meanwhile I made a decision. "I'll go nursing" I told Mum. "After all that is quite close to being a Doctor, and at least you can wear a uniform and sensible shoes!" She looked at me in amazement. "I think perhaps you should find out a bit more about nursing before you launch into it," she said. "It's not an easy job." But I had made up my mind.

We were now living in Melbourne, and the Royal Melbourne Hospital always looked romantic whenever we drove past, so I applied there immediately, but being just 17, had to wait until January of the next year, as trainees were not accepted under 17 years and 9 months of age. This left just enough time to fit the typing and shorthand course in between, so I launched into that at

Taylor's School of Commerce, to fill in the year. Even though I never intended to be a secretary in any sense, I always felt it necessary to apply myself to any task in hand as best I could, with the result that on completion of the course, I did so well I was offered a job at the College. "We know you're dedicated to nursing" said the College Principal, "but we'd like to offer you a job anyway just in case you change your mind." I got such a shock, and also feeling that though my shorthand wasn't too bad, if I had to take a letter I'd possibly have a fit, I declined. I often wondered afterwards just how different my life might have been if I had deviated at that point to a life of business, rather than one of helping to heal the sick. Unfortunately we will never know the answer to that, but I do believe it would not have been as likely that I would ever have ended up going to the Australian outback. The typing though has been forever useful, and I have never regretted having learnt that skill.

***

On January 14, 1964, I started nursing, and unexpectedly the first eight weeks were a nightmare. Despite the fact that we were placed in a beautiful old mansion in the glamorous and wealthy Melbourne suburb of Toorak for that time, and transported to and from the preliminary training school at the hospital every day by bus, I hated it. "Why had I embarked on this" I continually asked myself. The thought of enemas and bed baths haunted me, and I went home many an evening, as home was not too far from the living quarters, and wept on my mother's shoulder. Luckily I still did not neglect the studies, doing rather well despite my inner feelings, and when the time eventually came to look after real people, much to my amazement my whole approach changed and I adored it. Doing things for people who needed them done to solve their problems gave instant meaning to the previously odious tasks I had feared. I was starting to learn that things often do not turn out to be exactly as they appear at first, and that one should never give up on something too early.

Learning this lesson was invaluable when later I was faced with many new situations which were initially very difficult.

Being the dutiful minister's daughter, I was still attending church every Sunday and carrying out a routine prayer and Bible reading daily, with a sort of perfunctory obedience. I still believed one must do what God wanted, but didn't aspire to the born-again Christian theories, so as a result, I refused to participate in Nurses Christian fellowships and the like.

I continued on enjoying my nursing, and then began to feel that natural need for a romantic relationship. At school I had been quite fearful of the boys. One unfortunate lad had had the audacity to ask me for a second dance at my first school dance, whereupon I had gone all cold on him and ruined any further opportunities for friendship. Later I worked this out as being perhaps due to having no brothers, living at an all girls school, and having a mother who always seemed fearful of us getting wrongfully involved with the opposite sex. Anyway whatever it was, I was a very slow starter! One thing which did help in those days of hospital-based nursing programs where we all lived together in the nurses home, was that this provided a unique setting for camaraderie between colleagues in the same group, and enabled us to have social outings together with members of the opposite sex with less nervousness. For some, of course, there were also the parties in the young Resident doctor's quarters nearby, but due to the persistence of my above-mentioned shyness, I did not attend any of those parties; but I did admire many of the doctors from afar! I also had friends of both sexes at my local church, but none of the few males there seemed to fit the bill as a suitable partner for me, so I reluctantly decided to wait until the right person appeared.

At the end of nurse training came the usual celebratory ball. As I still had no-one special to ask, I took along someone who lived near my parents and whom I had met at their local church. He was studying psychology and managed to upset me by asking how many of us there, had to arrange a partner rather than having someone to take. I was not impressed with his using us as part of his research! Then along came all the 21st birthdays one after the other. For mine I decided I would go unaccompanied, invite all my male and female friends and acquaintances and dance with everyone. It was great, and I felt important and free, but I also knew that it wouldn't be so easy when I went to the other parties. Currently attending St Mary's Anglican Church North Melbourne, I commandeered a boy from there, and off I went to the first of my friends' formal coming-of-age. There I met a medical student from the Royal Melbourne who was at present dating that particular friend. She had been flirting with him for some weeks at the hospital, and suddenly there at her birthday party as her partner, he was asking me to go out with him.

I was appalled. How could he ask me out when he was partnering my best friend? I should have heard the warning bells then but was probably too naive. "I think this is quite inappropriate" I told him, but was secretly thrilled by the idea. The kernel of physical attraction sent shivers through me, but I suggested we wait until I returned to the Melbourne for my Staff Nurse year the following April.

***

Walking up the stairs to my first staff nurse ward placement he was suddenly in front of me. The old feeling of excitement shot through my stomach and I flushed red. A mumbled greeting and he was gone again. I could hardly work that day.

The next night he phoned and we went out. For some reason I tried to act as if this relationship was of no moment to me, and because I was not sure of how important he still was to my friend, I kept this alliance secret. I was also suddenly having quite a good time socially now in other areas, so decided to maintain this as a friendship only, and we mutually agreed that we should feel free to date others. Meanwhile, as I loved dancing, we did attend a couple of balls together, and went out for coffee quite a bit.

My mother was pleased when she heard of my friendship. A

trainee doctor for her daughter was just what she thought would be ideal. Despite her continued need of assistance in the home since her breakdown, she happily said if I married a Doctor she would just disappear into the woodwork and make no further demands on my time. I felt it was amazing that she should feel this way, as she had been quite negative about other boys who had shown some interest in me prior to this. Surprisingly I received no discouragement from any point, and when I finally confessed this relationship to my friend who had first gone out with him, even she was in favour. "He was always more your type than mine Audrey," she said warmly, and wished me all the best.

Time passed and my ward placement gave way to a stint in the Casualty department. I didn't mind this so much, but the roster there was to work me every Sunday on a PM shift. My male companion was a born again Christian, he had said. "So am I" I thought, but still didn't feel too comfortable with the terminology. As well as the other outings already mentioned, we had been going to church together on Sunday evenings, sometimes to my church St Mary's, and sometimes to his, St Jude's Carlton. The former was what I would call a high church atmosphere somewhat akin to Catholicism, which was not foreign to me as my mother had attended a convent in her youth and often spoke of Catholic philosophy. I felt comfortable with St Mary's, especially as they were not asking me if I was saved, which to me was Baptist theology. St Jude's however was quite into the 'Born again' bit, and this made me feel uncomfortable. Likewise Anglican, it was low church evangelical type, which was strange to me, my Dad being what my mother called a 'middle of the road' Anglican. This, she used to teach me, was the beauty of Anglicanism. It embraced all types of Christian philosophies from those who thought one needed a conversion experience, right through to those who thought we should never have left behind the incense and statues of Catholicism. I thought to myself, "evangelical Anglicanism is not for me." My companion recognised this and seemed keen to convert me, but I remained sceptical despite still being very attracted to him. I was also growing to love this man, but was not telling him about that.

The Sunday evening shifts brought to a climax what was probably bound to happen sooner or later. I suddenly saw less of my previously frequent escort, and one day the phone call came. "I've been going out steadily with someone else for some time" he said bluntly. A knife-like feeling went through me. I hung up, pushed past my mother, averting my eyes from her questioning gaze, and fled to the bedroom, where I threw myself down on the bed and sobbed uncontrollably. I could no longer see any point to it all.

CHAPTER 3 A NEW BEGINNING

Sydney 1968

I was depressed for most of the ensuing months following the break-up. Work was still interesting, God still somewhere in the maze, but life had lost its lustre. Little did I know that it was probably only then that I was ready to embrace a new lifestyle. I had decided some years before, to do midwifery wherever my now married sister happened to be living at the time. As she and her husband were buying a house in the Blue Mountains in NSW, I chose Crown Street Women's Hospital in Sydney. Leaving Melbourne behind for a while should help with the pain I thought.

Crown Street was quite different from the multi-storey cream brick of RMH. It was the oldest Midwifery training hospital in Australia, white painted stone walls, mostly only one or two storeys high, and situated within walking distance of the heart of Sydney. I had been to Sydney once before with my mother when I was about 14. We had greatly enjoyed the experience so I was looking forward to it. Besides, I could go to my sister's on days off, and we had been good friends since we had grown past the days of childhood jealousies.

My mother herself had been the oldest of three children, the younger two always seeming to gang up against her, so she had made it her plan, that when she married, she would have two girls one after the other, and they would be friends. By some stroke of good fortune she had had her two girls, and then managed to eventually help them to become friends, just as she had hoped.

Arriving in Sydney at last, the most fascinating aspect of the first few days in my new world, was the hemlines of our uniforms. At the Royal Melbourne we had worn them halfway down our calves, but here we were presented with miniskirts. The small, grey-headed home sister enquired, "Are your uniforms OK?" "Yes," I said tentatively, "but they are miles too short." She laughed loudly. "You should see the others", and that was that.

Settled into my new room in the nurse's home on the first night, there was an unexpected knock at the door, and I opened it to see two strangers smiling across at me. "We are members of the NCF or Nurses Christian Fellowship", they said, "and we wondered if you would like to come along to our meetings. We have them on Tuesday nights in the downstairs sitting room." I quickly made some excuse and somehow got rid of them from the door. As mentioned earlier, I didn't want any part of this sort of faith. However, I couldn't stop thinking about their visit. "How do you know you won't like it", I asked myself, "if you've never been to one of those meetings before?"

The next day we individually met the Matron of the hospital. She was a warm friendly lady who, zooming in on the fact that I was a minister's daughter, mentioned I might like to attend an Anglican Church near Kings Cross. This suggestion didn't really bother me, as I had wanted to find a place to worship. I thanked her and resolved to take her up on it.

Tuesday came and I was off duty in the evening. "Go down and see what it is like" I bullied myself, and before I knew it I was at the Nurses Christian Fellowship meeting. It was just as I had expected—a 'holy huddle', and by that I mean, they seemed to be grouped together, 'we know what you need and we're going to help you find it' sort of attitude, or that was how I perceived it. I sat it out but hated it, and vowed not to have any more to do with them. Later I discovered that they were very nice people, and my feelings were probably coloured by the fact that I did not understand where they were coming from. I also learnt afterwards, that the forces of evil can try to distract us from finding the truth, and were probably working hard right then to keep me in the dark.

Sunday dawned and I was off duty again. In the corridor I met one of the NCF girls. "Would you like to come with me to St John's Darlinghurst?" she asked kindly. This was the church Matron had suggested, so despite the enquirer being from that group I so disliked, I agreed to go with her that evening. To this day I do not recall what was said in the sermon that night. The service was a traditional Anglican one with which I was only too familiar, but something about the sermon was different. The minister was a small nuggety dynamic man, with jet-black hair and an infectious enthusiasm. "I've been going to church all my life," I said to him at the door, "and I've never before heard anyone preach like you." "That's interesting," he said. "How would you like to read this book", and he leaned over to a shelf behind him and offered me a small paperback. I took it home and sat up in bed. "By Searching" by Isabel Kuhn.

I read into the early hours, strangely fascinated by this girl's life story. Isabel had been a vivacious young medical student, enjoying ballroom dancing and all the other social trappings of her era, when suddenly she had become a born again Christian through a conversion experience. As a result of this she gave up some much-loved pastimes—reading secular literature, playing cards, and the beloved ballroom dancing being amongst them. I was astounded. I too loved ballroom dancing, and couldn't imagine that God would expect this kind of commitment.

The next week I took the book back. "I think that this is all a bit extreme", I told Mr Gook. Without missing a beat he took the book from my hand and replaced it with another. "Try this one" he said, "Basic Christianity" by John Stott. This author was an Anglican minister at All Soul's Langham Place in London. If he thought one needed a conversion experience I felt I just might be able to believe it. Meanwhile I wrote home to Mum and Dad. "Pray for me" I asked. "I'm going through a difficult time."

As I sped through the pages of John Stott's book I was nervous. I felt I was on the edge of something new and challenging, but I was also fearful of it. As I continued I came to a prayer, which one could say if one wanted to accept Jesus as one's Lord and Saviour. I had the overwhelming feeling that if I let this opportunity pass me by, I would never be given it again. I said the prayer and went to bed.

The next day I didn't feel any different. A troubled state of mind which had settled on me these past couple of weeks remained. Pacing up and down in our living quarters that evening I was still upset, so I did what my compulsive eating habits acquired at boarding school had led me to, and went to the pantry and had a large piece of bread, spread with beautiful grape jam, which seemed to be a Crown Street special. Instead of feeling better, I felt worse. It was now about 10.30 PM. I knew that down the corridor a small Asian nurse lived. I also knew that she was one of the Christians who went to the Nurses Christian Fellowship meetings, but she didn't seem as disturbingly zealous as the others. I crept up the corridor to her room and noted that the light was still shining under her door. I took a deep breath and knocked gently.

"Come in," said Judy with a questioning look. "I want to become a Christian," I blurted out before I lost the courage to say it. "I have this prayer in this book and I would like to say it in front of you." Understandingly she knelt down one side of the bed and gestured for me to do the same at the end, and I proceeded to read the prayer. Almost immediately after completing this, and following a short impromptu prayer from Judy, I left her, and went to bed. I slept soundly.

The wake-up call which we all received at 5.30 AM when we were rostered on an early shift, rocked me back into reality. I bounced out of bed. I felt different. Half an hour later sitting feeding a baby in the adoption nursery, my Fijian nursing companion looked intently across at me. "There is something different about you today," she said, "something spiritual". I was shocked. I knew that I was different, but I was amazed that she could see it, and was sure that she wouldn't have had time to be told about it by Judy. I found out later that some people seem to be very switched on to spiritual things, especially people of colour.

My new feelings were that I now automatically felt a love for my fellow human beings such as I had never before experienced. I also realised my own unworthiness to receive anything special from God, where before I had always felt that I was a pretty deserving person. Humility had taken over, and whilst I felt the need of God more than before, I somehow knew I now had the indwelling of the Holy Spirit promised by Jesus to his followers as a guiding force within me. I also felt that this was all I needed to live the kind of life the Bible always talks about—a life of service and love which, though sometimes traumatic, ultimately leads to an amazingly wonderful and otherwise unknown sense of fulfilment. It was lucky at this point that I did not know the extent of the traumas that lay ahead for me as I pursued this lifestyle, or I might not have so willingly embraced it. In retrospect though, even through the tough times, I have never regretted this decision, stumbled upon as if by chance, but so lovingly planned for all of us I believe, by a caring maker at the beginning of time. Despite my strong feelings of the spirit of God inside me, I did not then, nor since, speak in tongues, but still believe this is not mandatory for all Christians, but a gift given to some. My gifts were of other types, and I was quite comfortable with that.

***

With my new faith, life took on a whole new meaning. I even quite happily joined the 'holy huddle', and suddenly saw no division between the denominations of the Christian religion. I went to Baptist services and felt at home with them. Overwhelmingly I was sure that I had found the true purpose of life. We were here not for ourselves, but to serve God and our fellow man. Through this would come real happiness, and no longer would that feeling of no meaning cause me pain.

I sang to myself as I trotted along the streets on beautiful blue sky Sydney days, or sped joyously between the puddles while under an umbrella in the midst of heavy rainy downpours. "Why didn't you ever tell me what a wonderful life Christianity could provide?" I asked my mother and father, and then proceeded to earbash everybody I met about my new-found faith. Not that I wanted to ram it down their throats. I just knew what it had done for me, and wanted them to share it. No longer did I feel the need for a romance either, at least not at this stage. I felt ready now instead to take on whatever God had in mind.

CHAPTER 4 THE BUSH CHURCH AID SOCIETY

An Anglican missionary group committed to Outback Australia, THE BUSH CHURCH AID SOCIETY (B.C.A.) was first conceived on 26th May 1919, when 23 people attended a meeting in the Chapter House of St Andrew's Cathedral in Sydney to discuss the foundation of a society which could operate in all States, organise the resources of all Capital cities, and concentrate energy and service upon the neglected bush areas where men and women had ventured to find their fortune. Unfortunately many of the people to whom the society planned to minister, had found themselves in situations of great hardship, did not always make the money out of mining or pastoral holdings that they thought they would, or even if they did, sometimes became lonely and disillusioned in such sparsely populated and isolated country.

In the beginning the society had no resources, no office, only a burning desire to share the Gospel of Christ with outback people, and the firm conviction that God would provide, and so the Bush Church Aid Society was born. (Ref. "Those First Seventy Years"). In 1920 the first two missionaries went out, one to Wilcannia in the Diocese of Riverina, and the other to the Parish of Cobar in the Diocese of Bathurst.

As the years passed and more ministers went to new areas of outreach, B.C.A.'s concern for the whole person initiated an extension of the work into medical service. This was started in Ceduna with the opening of the first hospital in 1925. This hospital was replaced in 1931 and the medical work expanded into

Aboriginal areas with a hospital at Koonibba, and the Bishop Kirkby Memorial Hospital being built at Cook, and named for the first organising missioner S.J. Kirkby. The Flying Medical Service established in 1938, made servicing of the hospitals more efficient. The first flight out of Ceduna in a Fox Moth VH AAA was made by Alan Chadwick, the man who thirty years later was to fly a Beechcraft Baron over some of the same route when the B.C.A. Flying Medical Service was closed down, and the plane was handed over to its new owners, the Royal Flying Doctor Service of South Australia. This became the policy of the society—to pioneer and establish the answer to a need, and then to relinquish control of each enterprise when and if someone else, Government or otherwise, was willing to take it over. Then B.C.A. could spend their funds, mostly voluntary donations, on other new and needed ventures.

I first heard of B.C.A. at the age of 8. For some reason I was into collecting missionary moneyboxes, and simply added the little bark hut to my collection. As I was not very wealthy at the time, I put very little if any money into anything, with the consequence that four years later I received a letter from the new Victorian secretary John Stockdale, asking me if I intended to continue with my initial commitment, as I had been receiving the society newspaper, The Real Australian, and not contributing a penny for quite some time! I wrote back to explain that I was now only 12 years old, which I found out later when Mr Stockdale visited Ballarat, caused some amusement in the Victorian Office, and I was duly forgiven! I still did not know at that time that I would one day work for the society whose motto had become "Australia for Christ". Indeed as indicated earlier, at that time I would not have been really sure of quite what that meant. It was only now that I knew I could work for B.C.A. with a true understanding of its philosophy.

I pushed open the door to B.C.A. head office in Sydney and asked about the work. They were very keen for me to go as soon as my midwifery year was over, but I felt I needed to consolidate my obstetric knowledge, and knew my mother would not cope if I went away again so soon. I disappointed them by saying that it would probably be a year or so before I could join their outback staff, but I now knew my destiny was clear and no longer did I have any fear.

CHAPTER 5 GETTING READY

A new Christian is inevitably beset almost immediately by challenges to the faith, so it was really no surprise that just as I was learning to enjoy my new relationship with God and other believers, bad news came from Melbourne. My father had had a heart attack, and my mother was naturally upset. I tried to get some time off immediately to go home and see them, but Matron was not very co-operative, and I was forced to wait until my days off.

Finally home, I walked to the foot of his hospital bed. My father was dying. Despite this, visiting hours were still restricted, so I was only allowed a limited time. Reluctantly I left the hospital, and needing to return a key to the Verger's wife at St John's Toorak, where my father had been relieving when he had taken ill, I diverted there on my way home. A warm and friendly lady greeted me at the door, took the key, and enquired about my Dad. Tearfully I described his condition. She led me into the chapel, such a beautiful place at this oh-so-posh Melbourne church, and together we knelt to pray. Following this prayer together, somehow I knew immediately, that despite outward appearances, God was going to heal my father.

Dashing off home I arrived in time for a phone call from the Alfred Hospital. "Is that Mr Nixon's daughter". "Yes," I replied. The voice continued. "Your father's condition has deteriorated and we have put him on the dangerously ill list. As a result you may come in any time." I hung up and instead of being distressed by this news, I danced around the kitchen. Somehow I knew the answer to our prayer was still valid. I was just happy that the visiting was no longer restricted. Basket packed I took off again for the hospital, and sat gratefully by my Dad.

Sure enough he did get better, well enough to resume work for at least another six years, and I had experienced my first personal miracle, and my first example of Romans Chapter 8 Verse 28 which is now my favourite verse in the Bible. "All things work together for good for those who love God and are called according to His purpose." Taking back the key, and meeting the verger's wife that day, had all fitted into place for a good outcome. I returned to Sydney, my new faith having been tried and not found wanting.

The Midwifery exams were coming up, and in deference to God's teaching on our need to have one day of rest each week, I decided not to study on Sundays. Never before had I taken such a risk, especially for exams on a Monday morning! To my amazement and delight, when my results came in, they were the best I had ever achieved. It seemed to me that God had honoured my sacrifice, and at the same time blessed me with wonderful Sundays of worship, fellowship, and true refreshment, due to the break from the usual responsibilities.

The year in Sydney completed, it was now time to go home again. Back in Melbourne however, life proved to be more difficult than I had expected. My parents were uncomfortable with my new philosophy, and my mother in particular seemed to misunderstand me more than usual. I had planned to live at home and travel to work each day to my new job at the Royal Women's Hospital. However when I tried to do this with the inevitable shift work and no car of my own, I found it very difficult and decided to move into the nurses' home. This was not appreciated by the family, my mother especially being very disappointed at my leaving home again so soon, but I felt I had no other option.

Life at the Royal Women's was tough but educational. I didn't know then that later in the outback I was going to need some of those very lessons learnt, to prevent an obstetric disaster. I also did Infant Welfare with leave of absence from the Women's, and that too was vital for my still unknown future responsibilities. I now attended church at St Jude's Carlton. What a strange coincidence, and how I now loved that church. I learned that my previous love had gone to New Zealand with one girl, and come back with another. I could actually see the funny side of it all.

I approached the Society again, officially applied for the work, and was accepted without question. The three B.C.A. hospitals in South Australia, namely Cook, Tarcoola, and Coober Pedy, were now fully staffed, so it was decided that after relieving at each place for the girls to have a short break, I, with another B.C.A. girl from Sydney, would then go to Laverton in Western Australia, and work there for two years lent to the Government Hospital. The die was cast.

I had made some wonderful friends at St Jude's who were to support me from afar throughout my outback work. It was St Jude's who took official responsibility for praying and keeping in contact with me, and it was they who circulated my prayer letters. The minister at the time, David Binns, was a most loving person, and my Valedictory service held there was very special. Still, however, things were not well on the home front. In the long run Mum supported me one hundred percent, but it wasn't until after I left for the outback that she came to terms with my vocation.

Luckily within me I knew my decision was correct, and managed to ride through the dissent, supported by my newfound faith.

The time arrived for my departure. Packed and ready, Mum and Dad saw me off at Spencer Street railway station. They were sad, and I was apprehensive, and even though I knew by now that God would surely be going with me, the way ahead suddenly looked very scary indeed.

CHAPTER 6 A DESERT EXPERIENCE

South Australia–March, 1971

Loneliness was my only emotion as I stepped from the train. Loneliness that gnawed into my stomach and drained the feeling from my body, until I wanted to move away from it and return to reality. Reality as I had always known it, at home with the family, or even as a child at boarding school. Nothing had ever felt this empty.

My eyes scanned the flat, treeless landscape, the endless nothingness and unimaginable silence of a faraway place. Nullarbor, I thought, it's a good name. A single row of houses broke the monotony, but even they did not do much to remove the immediate sense of isolation. I still firmly believed that I had answered God's call to work in outback Australia for B.C.A., and that He would instruct me and show me the way to go, but right now my legs felt numb.

"Is that all the luggage you have?" I turned quickly at the sound of an unknown voice. A pleasant-looking round-faced man smiled cheekily. He put out his hand and shook mine warmly. "I'm Brian," he said. "Welcome to Cook."

Taking the suitcases from my side he settled them into the boot, and then helped me into his dust-covered car. Starting the engine he said cheerily. "Might as well take you straight to the hospital. Pam and Ruth are waiting for you there."

The hospital was like a large old-fashioned country homestead, with a verandah almost all the way around. Situated at the far end of the previously noted row of houses, it seemed to me to be protecting the settlement from the endlessness of the horizon. It was March and the weather was decidedly warm. Luckily, I loved the heat.

Beside the hospital was a square tank, painted white and inscribed in red...IF YOU'RE CROOK COME TO COOK on one side, and...OUR HOSPITAL NEEDS YOUR HELP GET SICK! on the other. In between was a map of South Australia, with COOK QUEEN CITY OF THE NULLARBOR written on it in the same red paint. The humour of this monument helped ease my discomfort.

Cook was strictly a railway town, halfway across the Transline. This term meant the TransAustralian Railway line, which runs from east to west, from Port Pirie, South Australia to Kalgoorlie in Western Australia. One could connect with this line from Sydney on the Indian Pacific train, or from Adelaide on the Transcontinental, and travel right across to Perth, the capital of W.A. Cook was therefore almost in the middle of the Nullarbor Plain. This stretch was said to be the longest straight stretch of railway in the world. Travelling in the train it had certainly felt like it. As the unfamiliar terrain had passed the windows, all one could see was flat earth, small scrubby bushes, and endless deep blue sky. The landscape had sung its own song, in harmony with the sound of the speeding train, but I hadn't felt bored, it was fascinating. Nevertheless, now off the train, and on this very flat land itself, uncertainty was uppermost in my mind.

Pam, I soon discovered, was Brian's wife, and Ruth, an English girl, my co-worker for the forth-coming month. They both made me feel very welcome, and showed me where to put my things. My room was on the end of the building just inside the built-in verandah door. The smell was distinctive but did not remind me of anything which I had previously encountered. It seemed to be a combination of dust, heat, and some unknown essence which much later I came to love. The room was bright and airy with a window on the left-hand side, looking out to the small barren garden and the Nullarbor beyond. A pretty pink bedcover gave a flavour of homeliness, and the furniture was of a pale lacquered wood which was quite attractive.

Pam and Brian Sard lived next door, inhabitants of this faraway place with the compliments of the Australian Postal Department. Brian was a P.M.G. Technician, and Pam ran the Post Office. Pam, a very athletic girl, had been a state women's cricketer when younger, and still looked very fit. She and Brian had one little boy Brendan, whom I was yet to meet. I discovered quite quickly that these two people were our real friends, always ready to help, and also to share in our outreach. Pam had been converted to Christianity as a result of the enticement of Maud's cakes! More about Maud later. The town consisted of little else except a store, hall, school, twenty houses, and of course, the hospital, the latter being the intended workplace for my first assignment. Pam made a few friendly comments and then took off home to other duties. Unpacked, I joined Ruth in the lounge.

I was soon to learn that this six-bed hospital was divided into living quarters one end and wards the other, that most of the work was outpatient oriented, and inpatients were rare. This latter point was probably a good thing as generally we were on duty 24 hours a day, making the care of inpatients quite tiring. Any serious illnesses though, were not kept at this little outpost, as there was no resident Doctor. The work at Cook was totally foreign to me, but I hoped that I would settle in quickly.

The next morning I got up to find Ruth preparing breakfast which we ate at the table in the kitchen. After polishing off cereal, toast and Vegemite, she opened the Bible as we sipped our tea. "We always have a reading and prayer after breakfast" she said. It sounded good to me, as I was still feeling decidedly inadequate. We read and prayed, and as always when one doesn't feel like praying but continues on and does it anyway, I felt the comfort.

Prior to breakfast Ruth had already listened to the Flying Doctor Service morning session on the two-way radio. This, she explained to me, was an important part of our work, firstly to keep in touch with flying doctor happenings, and secondly a cheaper way to get advice when and if we needed it. Each outpost had a call sign which was used to make the connection. From Cook, one held down the button of the handpiece and spoke "9 Romeo Oscar, 9 Romeo Oscar." "Go ahead Ruth" came the doctor's friendly voice. "We need some advice on a patient who came on the train yesterday etc. etc." There were four sessions a day. Outside of these we could always use the telephone.

Despite the prayers, I was still feeling that the settling in bit was going to be a lot more difficult than I had previously supposed. Breakfast over and the dishes done, Ruth was off to the local primary school to teach Religious Instruction, or R.I. as it was known. She had prepared the previous day, and offered to take me along. I was grateful to see how it was done because I knew that this would be part of my work, and was acutely aware that I had never done it before. Following my conversion in Sydney, I had had little opportunity to teach Sunday School, as shift work often precluded regular commitments, and care of my mother took up a lot of my spare time when I was at home in Melbourne.

Even though my faith had grown and matured a lot since that exciting time in Sydney, the difficulties at home had made me less confident again. The spiritual responsibilities of my forthcoming job were a decided worry for me. The B.C.A. fellows had said, "You'll be all right. You love the Lord, and basically you are going out there to nurse." They didn't really mention all the other things. The pattern was that the two nurses would take it in turns to cover the hospital workload: nursing one fortnight, cooking and housework the other. Then there was the shared tasks of spiritual outreach which in Cook included Sunday school and church on Sundays, kids club Mondays, Bible Study group on Tuesdays, and Religious Instruction at the school on Thursday mornings. With no resident minister of religion, we were it. We climbed into the little blue-grey VW and roared off down the dirt road. The sky was still as blue as yesterday, and a cloud of dust billowed behind us.

Sitting at the back of the class I listened panic-stricken to Ruth competently teaching. She also led the children in a string of Bible songs which not only did they know exceptionally well but seemed to enjoy immensely. "How could I ever do this?" I asked myself. "Surely I had made the wrong move coming all the way out here." I confided as much to Ruth a little later. She looked at me with some sympathy and said, "You'll cope, I had to."

At least I had been trained for the nursing part, or had I? This was mostly casualty type, but as mentioned before there was no local doctor! The flying doctor visited only once a month for a clinic. In between one simply had to look after everything that turned up on the doorstep, as if one were the local G.P. As described, the doctor could always be contacted via the phone or two-way radio, and anything too big for the nurses to handle was flown out to Port Augusta, but right at this moment everything looked big to me.

My cooking expertise was also not the most reliable. My sister had lovingly furnished me with a P.W.M.U. Cookery book as a parting gift. Inscribed on the inside cover were the words, "To assist you in the middle of nowhere." I was feeling I'd need plenty of assistance.

"Are you coming?" Ruth's voice filtered through my tumbling thoughts. The classes, senior and junior were over and she was making her way to a small house to the left of the two-storey school building. "Where are we going?" "To the usual reward for frazzled R.I. teachers" grinned Ruth. "Katy always rescues us with a cup of tea." What a wonderful idea.

Katy Briffa was the wife of Paul, the current headmaster of Cook Primary School, and mother of their three children. Paul and Katy were an Italian couple more recently from Adelaide, and Paul had decided to take on the job at Cook without a clear idea of exactly where it was geographically. The isolation had therefore been quite a shock to them both, but they seemed to be bearing up well. Katy was also a schoolteacher, and I warmed to her straight away. She had a lovely smile, blond hair piled up on her attractive head, and was apparently a whizz at home-made pasta. That was something to look forward to. "How did you both go today?" she bubbled. "I didn't do anything," I admitted ruefully, "I left it all to Ruth." "Good idea" laughed Katy. "Plenty of time for everything soon enough". Tea over we said our goodbyes, and roared off home to a lunch of bought meat pie and veg—the easiest thing to get at short notice, and, I was to find out, usual for Thursday lunch after R.I. My mind was still working overtime. "Would I ever learn all I needed to, to feel comfortable in this new and different world?" I guessed I would have to just wait and see.

CHAPTER 7 THE FIRST LESSONS

We sat down after lunch and Ruth automatically brought out her needlework. "Would you like to start by handling the cooking etc. and move gradually into the medical side of things?" she asked kindly. I agreed immediately to this suggestion. I wasn't too sure what I was going to cook, but it couldn't be too difficult. Ruth continued: "We usually have the same breakfast of cereal, toast and tea, and our main meal at lunch. Then in the evening can be something of a snack. There are lots of cookery books in the kitchen. You can experiment all you like. We also cook for inpatients of course, and the Doctor and Pilot on Doctor's day, but that isn't for another two weeks so you'll be right into it by then. Anyway we help one another when necessary, so don't feel you can't ask me when you need a hand."

When the evening mealtime came near, I moved into the kitchen. Ruth had already suggested something simple which I found to my relief I had no trouble producing. So far the stove was the most comforting facet of my new world. It was a large slow combustion, a vivid reminder of my childhood. I just knew I was going to enjoy it. The thought of cooking for inpatients, however, still terrified me, and doctor's day was a definite worry.

The kitchen was plain but serviceable, sink on one side, stove the other, cupboards around the walls, and a table in the middle. Most foods available at home could be found here, except that fresh milk and meat were only obtained once a week. We usually drank powdered milk in between, definitely not my favourite. We froze a week's supply of meat, taking something out each day for lunch. We ate our evening meal in the lounge room on the dining table, the usual eating place I discovered later, for both lunch and dinner. The lounge was very homely, a wood heater in the centre of the outside end and a narrow window on either side of that. Out the windows you could see the extent of our back yard—seventy miles of it, flat, dry, and no flowers! Years later I was drawn to and bought a house with the same configuration in the lounge room of fireplace and narrow window on each side. It reminded me of Cook and I felt at home with that reminder. Back at Cook the two-way radio sat on a table under the left-hand window, with lounge chairs on either side of the room, while the dining table was the other end nearest the door. Ruth's voice interrupted my thoughts. "We usually read the Bible and pray again after tea" she announced. Again this was no problem for me, as I needed this badly. Besides I had not known when to fit in my daily time of prayer and Bible reading with God yet…perhaps I would set the alarm for a little earlier in the morning and fit it in before getting breakfast. Prayers over we cleaned up the dishes together, and then out came Ruth's sewing again. I realised this was the Cook habit, as Pam had popped in earlier and she had her knitting. I would have to get myself some occupational therapy or I could feel very out of it here! I contented myself with starting a letter to home as I had received a telegram earlier. "Hope the trip was good. Thinking of you. Love Mum and Dad." What on earth was I going to say to them? Tell them everything I decided…just how it is.

***

The alarm clock shocked me into the next day and I remembered my resolve to get up and have a quiet time. I crept to the kitchen and revved up the remaining hot coals to see if I could boil the kettle. Successful, I crept back along the veranda trying not to wake Ruth whose room I had to pass on the way. As at home, I climbed back into bed with my hot coffee and Bible, and opened to the day's scripture reading and commentary. As always it was comforting and I was pleased that my plan had worked. I was to get breakfast today, so toileted and dressed I returned to the kitchen where as I toasted the bread on the hot coals from the end of a long toasting fork [very reminiscent of my childhood again], I could hear Ruth listening to the two-way radio. I had survived two whole days and day three was on the way!

Dishes done and floor swept, Ruth and I set off for the store and post office in the VW. This I discovered was to be a weekday ritual. The mail we collected ourselves, and there always seemed to be something to pick up at the store, or the station, or just someone to say hello to. The people were very friendly, and I felt immediately welcomed by everyone. Pam was at her post stamping and bagging the letters and promised to see us later. She usually popped in for afternoon tea and a chat most days after her work was finished.

Back at the hospital with some medical work and morning tea and lunch over, I soon saw that most afternoons were devoted to preparing for those spiritual responsibilities listed last chapter. The kid's club held on Monday nights was to me a complete unknown. This was for the older children of the town, both boys and girls, and they all seemed to enjoy coming. We began with some obviously well known Christian choruses sung with gusto, then a very innovatively presented Bible story. Finally games outside, floodlit by a light on the wall of the hospital, and then we walked all the children home. Despite my initial fears, I found it very fulfilling.

Adult Bible study on Tuesday nights was also very rewarding for us. Not many of the people came, mainly only Pam and Brian, but this was still a time when we could share God's word together and build up our faith. Another night once a month, the hospital auxiliary met to make things for selling. Now I knew if I had been staying at Cook I would have had to get into this, but secretly I was rather glad I wasn't, as this was not really my thing.

Thursday night was battinton at the local hall. This was a

hospital fund-raising event and we always baked a cake. The people who came paid for the privilege and a good game was had by all. In a town with very little entertainment available, battinton was a definite drawcard. For the uninitiated this was a cross between badminton and table tennis I thought, the net high as in beachball games, and racquets used to hit the shuttlecock back and forth over it. This game was good fun.

Saturday night was a visit to the butcher on the train as there was no butcher in the town. Wouldn't have been practical I suppose, as there wouldn't have been any cattle to kill, so the butcher came to us every Saturday night on the Tea and Sugar train. Everyone climbed up onto the train and bought their meat as in any other butcher shop, though this one was quite unique as it travelled up the line to all the little places along the way. After the butcher, evening meal, and dishes were out of the way, it was over to the Sards to play cards! My only problem with Saturday nights was that if I was to do the Sunday sermon for our service on Sunday afternoon, I had to have it finished by then, as well as my Sunday school lesson prepared for Sunday morning. Nevertheless playing 'Joe' every Saturday night was very relaxing and worth putting the effort in beforehand to reap the reward. You might be saying at this point where was all the medical work? It was really quite fragmented. People came by goods train from the small camps up and down the line, and the local people dropped in when they needed any help. Sometimes we were busy with the occasional inpatient, but generally life was quite domestic except for Doctors day (more about that a little later). We also flew out anything serious or surgical. Just as well, I don't think I would have liked to attempt untrained scalpel use! The plane was arranged by phone call or radio contact with the flying Doctor, the pilot and a nurse usually came, or if no nurse was available, one of us went with the patient. I was always happy to go because I loved flying, but for those who didn't it was not a favourite thing. At night the airstrip was not lit up, so if we needed to evacuate anyone, all the townspeople with cars came and parked beside the strip with their lights on full beam, and this provided sufficient illumination for both landing and taking off. This scene was always quite dramatic and a source of much discussion the next day in the town.

Washing and ironing, for the hospital as well as personal, was a routine weekly event, as the accounts were a monthly one. I guess the routine would have upset some people, but I loved that aspect. Would have been reminiscent of boarding school I suppose.

***

Before I knew it, Thursday had come around again, and this time it was my turn to try R.I. I had always thought I liked small children until I did my stint at the Royal Children's Hospital in Melbourne. There I discovered that it could be difficult to get them to do what was necessary, and for the whole three months there, I never seemed to master this. Now here I was, confronted with the same problem. It was only later that I learnt that oh-so-valuable lesson. When God plans to teach us something He repeatedly confronts us with the lesson until we have learnt it. Coping with children was to be one such lesson for me.

The children of Cook were not markedly different from children anywhere else, except that they were a mixture of Aboriginal and white Australian children. This however, did not seem to be a problem here as they appeared to get on remarkably well together. I soon found that the real difficulty was the universal one, that children at school in a religious instruction class could be absolutely beautiful or positively obnoxious. Competence in the teacher was of paramount importance. I was glad nobody knew just how little experience I had behind me.

With my carefully prepared lesson clutched in one hand, I entered the junior school classroom. With the exception of one rather taller-looking boy, these children were delightful. Being already very used to this kind of teaching, they seemed to soak up the Bible story. It was the taller boy who brought my so far controlled teaching debut to a crisis point. He suddenly jumped up out of his seat, making faces and laughing at everything that was said. I tried to control him verbally, then by ignoring him, but all to no avail. Before I realised what I had done, the chalk duster in my hand had come down on his shoulder with a whack!

It was not a hard hit, and it did bring the disturbance to an instant halt, but I was horrified. What made things even worse was that the duster mark remained clearly outlined on his jumper, my initial feeble attempts to remove it made impossible by the fact that every effort in this regard only served to accentuate my misdemeanour. I was relieved to move on to the seniors upstairs which luckily went uneventfully.

The classes ended, I literally flew next door. Katy laughed out loud. "Is that all you did to him," she said to me. "You should have seen him when I was trying to teach him. "Some of the swearwords he used in my class I'd barely heard before. I don't think a little tap on the back will affect that boy."

Well at least it was over for me for another fortnight. The VW transported me swiftly home the short distance to the hospital and Ruth also reassured me. Fortunately the Sunday school lessons were much less traumatic. At least these children came voluntarily, or with their parent's encouragement, to hear the Christian message. I enjoyed it immensely, my little group of wide-eyed youngsters drinking in every fascinating detail. If only R.I. could be a little more like that.

I noticed soon enough that it was not only the children here who appeared to be totally devoid of racist feelings. In Cook, it appeared to me anyway, there was complete integration of white and black, both living successfully in the same kind of houses, husbands doing the same kind of jobs, and no animosity even in the schoolground. The only sad part was, that in order to achieve this harmony, the Aboriginals seemed to have given away their culture completely. What a price to pay!

My first Doctor's day dawned with the usual blue sky and bright sunshine. "Does it ever rain here?" I asked Ruth in wonderment. "Not very often" she responded with a grin. "We only get about 4–6 inches the whole year, and every summer we often get the State's highest temperature. Our rival is Maree, but we nearly always beat them." It certainly had been hot each day but I was thoroughly enjoying it. I had always had a different thermostat, but had to admit I hated the cold. "It gets very cold here in winter" Ruth went on brightly. "Bright sunny days mostly, but cool with very cold nights". Definitely the extremes of the desert I mused, and appreciated the need for the wood-burning heater in the lounge room. But getting back to the heat, I had already discovered that even the summer hot days in Cook were cooled each evening by the 'Doctor'. Not the flying one of course, but the name given to the cool breeze coming seventy miles from the sea, south of the Nullarbor each night. "Nothing like that at Maree" quipped Ruth.

The sunsets and sunrises were also indescribable. With no buildings intervening, the landscape was completely viewed in all God's creative beauty, and the stars at night were definitely something else. If I wasn't so worried about everything I thought, I could almost enjoy this place…but no. TODAY IS DOCTORS DAY AND I AM STILL TERRIFIED.

I had spent all the day before preparing the meals and goodies which seemed to be the pattern for entertaining the flying doctor. Later he told me there was no way he would ever keep his figure having always to show appreciation for the culinary efforts put in by all the nurses on the way around the clinics. Normally we wore ordinary clothes both domestically and medically in this place, but today Ruth dressed in her white nurse's uniform to assist the doctor, and I rechecked the morning tea things for the hundredth time or so it felt.

"They arrive at 10" Ruth had told me, "and patients come from miles up and down the line either side of Cook, as well as from among the locals." Appointments made and clinic in readiness, even down to brilliantly polished floors, done by us of course, the place looked spotless. Beds had also been made in one of the two only four bed wards of the hospital, for the doctor and pilot who would stay overnight, and leave after breakfast the next morning for the next clinic. I was not a very good housekeeper either, legacy of boarding school and a mother not so well for many years I suppose, but I had been cleaning kitchen and bathrooms etc. since my arrival and was getting quite good at it I thought. "Where is the airstrip?" I had asked Ruth. "I imagined everyone came to Cook by train". Ruth had taken me out the backdoor of the hospital. "Right there" she said pointing to an area not much less barren than the rest of the terrain and almost no distance from where we were standing. "The plane then taxis right up to the back door. Very handy eh?" I would just have to see that I decided with a giggle.

The sound of a plane overhead brought me back to reality with a bang and I felt sick inside again. It's only a man after all and he can't eat me if his dinner isn't cooked properly. I honestly remember very little of Richard, as he left and was replaced by Byron not long after I started, but I knew that he had a reputation for very good medical skills, a necessity for the variety of work with which the Flying Doctor could be confronted. In my nervousness I hoped he wouldn't take too much notice of me. The plane was a twin engine Cessna, white, with Royal Flying Doctor Service of South Australia clearly inscribed on the side. It roared up to the back door just as Ruth had described, doctor and pilot jumped out, and my first doctor's day was underway.

***

The next morning as we turned our backs to prevent the dust from getting in our eyes, the plane rolled away towards take-off. It was over and I had survived. I had not had to participate at all in the clinic which seemed to run very smoothly. The pilot had sat in the lounge all day and more or less minded his own business. Meal times and morning and afternoon teas had floated by with me in some kind of a dream, serving on automatic pilot as it were and getting through with a minimum of discomfort. The pilot had even helped with the dishes. I thought "How nice". Richard had said a couple of things to me, but must have decided he wasn't going to interfere too much with the new kid on the block, for which I was grateful.

Returning to routine, my culinary skills had quite a workout in my month with Ruth. I tried a series of different recipes in the beautiful oven, and appreciated my mother's oft-spoken view that there was nothing like a wood stove. My only real problem was my first attempt at breadmaking which, due to the addition of water which was a little too hot, came out of the oven flat and hard. Needless to say that effort ended up in the incinerator at the back of the hospital! The medical side of things continued on as usual. Ruth handled most of it, and what I didn't know I learnt from her, and the medical textbooks on hand, as I went.

Although Ruth worked hard at whatever had to be done, and showed me as much as she could, and Pam and Brian next door were very supportive, I still felt very strange.

The first month seemed to pass quite quickly and Carol, Ruth's usual co-worker returned. I only had to work with her a few days, as Ruth, being English, did not have many local places she could visit in her break, so did not stay away very long. When she returned I was on the move again, this time to Tarcoola. I wasn't sorry to leave.

CHAPTER 8 NEXT STOP TARCOOLA

"Barry will be arriving at Cook in a day or so and will happily drive you to Tarcoola," Carol told me. Not another stranger was my immediate thought. Barry Rainsford was the B.C.A. minister stationed at Coober Pedy, 187 kilometres north of Tarcoola. Coober Pedy was an opal-mining town currently with approximately 4000 inhabitants, but it was not Barry's only pastoral responsibility. His need to regularly visit the rest of his 'flock' in places like Cook and Tarcoola, plus all the numerous sheep stations in between, enabled him to be a perfect means of transport for people like me. Also I was now beginning to realise what being part of the B.C.A. family really meant.

I was only to spend two weeks at Tarcoola, another railway town down the track towards Port Pirie, and then travel north to Coober Pedy to finish my round of relieving. Ruth, Carol, Pam, and Brian, gathered to say goodbye. I realised I had already become attached to all of them, but I was nevertheless now looking forward to moving on.

The road to Tarcoola was rough, dusty, and full of potholes. Before my time in these remote places was over I was to experience many roads such as this. It brought back the childhood trips around country Victoria, except that this was even more remote.

Maud and Heather came out to welcome us. Another homestead-like hospital confronted me, but this one was not so close to the railway line. I realised I was already becoming attached to the trains. After all I mused; they are our lifeline in these parts. The main thing that fascinated me here was the presence of a real Sturt Desert Pea beside the driveway. This was South Australia's floral emblem, striking red in colour with a jet-black blob in the centre of each bloom. There are actually some flowers on the Nullarbor I thought. What a fascinating plant, and to think it just grew up there all by itself. Later when I went to W.A. I was to see carpets of Australian wildflowers, which seemed to appear from nowhere after the rare patches of rain, but never again would I see a flower as vivid and unusual as this. I was entranced, and thoroughly enjoyed trapping its colour and uniqueness on a photographic slide, which was shared with many ardent B.C.A. supporters when I eventually returned home.

Barry introduced me to the Tarcoola nurses, but I still felt very strange. Heather left for her break the next day, and Barry, promising cheerfully that he would be back for me in a fortnight, also went his way. Maud and I were left.

Tarcoola was run similarly to Cook, so I knew next morning that housework would be on the agenda. Although as already intimated, not my favourite occupation, I set about mopping floors etc. with as much enthusiasm as I could muster. Maud was a household name along the transline. During her many previous years at Cook she had become renowned for her fantastic culinary abilities, not to mention her amazing skills of being able to produce a magnificent garden of vegetables and fruit trees in the middle of the desert. It was Maud's cakes that had attracted Pam to Christianity, and over the years Maud had indeed served well. She had retired from Cook, but when B.C.A. were unable to staff Tarcoola, she and Heather agreed to come out to keep the place open.

The medical work here was pretty sparse, and I was blessed with the only thing needing my attention being a burnt ankle, a similar injury to one I had watched being dealt with only the day before by Heather before she left. I was well aware, even in the desolation of my current state, that the Lord was providing.

The ministry provided by the girls in Tarcoola was very similar to Cook: Sunday school, Church Services, R.I. etc. Again I helped where I could and tried to be as confident as possible despite my ever present and continuing unease.

When Heather and Maud had both returned from their respective breaks, Barry collected me and stage three was on the way. Again I wasn't sad to leave.

CHAPTER 9 COOBER PEDY HERE I COME

Barry was an excellent travelling companion so the trip north was quite entertaining. A man with a very dry sense of humour, and a true Christian kindliness, he immediately won his way into my life. I recognised that here was a true friend. Barry was married to Jenny, whom I discovered when we reached Coober Pedy was also a beautiful person, not only in nature but physically as well. They had two children and an effective ministry to all the non-Catholic Christians resident in C.P. (the Catholics having their own priest that is). After the loneliness of Cook and Tarcoola, I recognised the advantage of a minister in the town. Something we all take for granted at home.

As Barry's car valiantly transported us over the now expected rough and unmade roads, we talked, in between me hopping out intermittently to open and close property gates. This was cattle country, and it was unforgivable to neglect the proper performance of the gate routine. At intervals we visited property homesteads. The families we met were incredibly hospitable, and plied us with all sorts of homemade goodies which were not too good for the figure. I should mention here that my figure had always been a problem. Boarding school where one was made to eat when one wasn't hungry and denied food when one was, had managed to very efficiently turn me into a foodaholic. Later in life the conquering of this was also to be a lesson learnt, but as yet it was still a problem which was to beset me throughout my outback career.

Coober Pedy was like no other place I had ever seen or imagined. Arid undulations dotted with piles of rubble I was later to discover were non back-filled drill holes. As these were not fenced or marked with danger in any way, how many unwanted or unaware Coober Pedy citizens ended up down one of those holes, never to be found or missed, was anybody's guess. This was a tough town. As we drove in I noted the swirls of dust as cars and trucks careered around the dirt roads. I soon learned that to live in Coober Pedy meant to eat, breathe and become encapsulated by dust. The hospital corridors were thick with it every morning, usually with a small cliff face along each skirting board. As you lifted the quilt off your bed you could smell it. I had been in the outback for all of about six weeks, and at this point I couldn't imagine that I was ever going to like it. I definitely underestimated the power and planning of God.

Anne and Shirley were the two B.C.A. nurses in charge at the Coober Pedy Medical Centre, as it was known. Neither of them wanted to go away for a break, so they suggested that I might just like to give them a hand for the two weeks planned. I did my best to do this for them as I quickly realised that two nurses in this busy place was no longer enough. It had been okay at the beginning when the town was only small, but now it was booming, and medical services were constantly in demand. There was a significant number of Christians in the town as well, which was such an encouragement after the loneliness of the other two areas.

The hospital mainly catered for outpatients, approximately 80 or more per day! Chest infections, burns and lacerations, plus all the things faced by a local GP at home, as well as those medical problems peculiar to a full-on mining town environment, poured in the front door of the hospital day and night. Anne and Shirley had it very well organised—clinic times, sterilising of equipment and supplies, delivering babies and so on. The townspeople had also created an ambulance service to collect accident cases which were not all that infrequent. The ambulance crew, Ross and Iris McArdle and helpers where needed, did a wonderful job of transporting the critically injured to the hospital, even to the point of bringing people up out of narrow mineshafts strapped to a stretcher to prevent any worsening of possible spinal injuries. Involved in one of the early rescues carried out in this manner, Anne had received a bravery award. I couldn't imagine that I was ever going to be able to function as adequately as these girls did. How often we underestimate God's willingness and power to assist and teach us.

The girls were also the local vets, even treating a snake for pneumonia. Don't think I would fancy that I thought to myself, and secretly admired their versatility.

Doctor's day here was once a week, which was quite understandable considering the volume of work. The airstrip was some distance out of town, so the pilot would buzz the hospital and then one of us would drive out and pick them up.

The fellowship of the Christians in Coober Pedy was very well organised. Church on Sunday in the little Catholic dugout we shared was quite special, and the Sunday school very well patronised. Sunday afternoon was always a chat session on the two-way radio with the other two B.C.A. hospitals. This I really enjoyed as I had already met them all and felt at home with them now. Coober Pedy hospital's call sign was '9 Sierra Foxtrot Papa'. Amid my ever-present inadequacies, I was finding there were some fascinating aspects of outback life.

Most of the houses in town were underground, but the hospital and vicarage opposite were above ground as at home, and so were the shops. It was quite a big town with a drive-in picture theatre, hotels, and clubs etc. As always the heat was ever present, so those with above ground homes needed air conditioners which were mostly water-cooled models.

The dugout homes varied in their complexity, from simple cave-like dwellings with minimal basic furnishings, to sumptuous, carpeted cave-mansions, with all the modern conveniences of gas stoves, refrigerators, built-in kitchen cupboards etc. One home even boasted a fully tiled underground swimming pool! The houses were normally formed by digging out earth from the side of a hill, therefore the front rooms would have windows giving natural light, while the rooms further back would only have light coming in from the air shaft which was made through the limestone roof to the top of the hill outside. Some dim light would come through this in the daytime, but as usually the rooms back further were the bedrooms, one could imagine inadvertently sleeping in without the sunshine to wake you, unless an alarm clock was used. The greatest thing about dugout homes was that they were very cool in the intense outback heat. Also if you wanted to extend, you simply got in the bulldozer and went a little further into the hillside. The other less frequent but equally possible advantage was the chance of coming across a seam of opal while you were building your house, and becoming a millionaire overnight. Now, that was something worth trying for.

Water in the town was supplied by the desalination plant, so, as with Cook, where water was brought in by train, this was quite a costly item.

Bill McDougall was a good friend to the girls, much as Brian Sard had been at Cook, and Bill provided an outlet every now and again by inviting us to his dug-out for dinner. There he would cook on his two Primus stoves, and after the meal we would play darts. It was good fun and Bill was a gem.

The fortnight went quickly. Before I knew it I was leaving again. I was happy.

CHAPTER 10 BEGINNING THE REAL TASK

Laverton was an old gold-mining town 360km north of Kalgoorlie. I had little knowledge of what to expect. All I knew was that this was to be my permanent position, probably for at least the next two years. I flew up there with the Kalgoorlie branch of The Royal Flying Doctor Service, and when I presented my two large suitcases to be loaded on to the plane, the pilot quipped. "You mean you are really going to stay up there for two years! You must be off your head." I laughed at him, but inside that feeling to which I had become extraordinarily used in the preceding weeks was bubbling away. I didn't tell him about it.

The trip was exciting. I had never before travelled in such a small plane. Always a person who had loved flying, I was ecstatic. The twin-engine Cessna zoomed over more desolate country, this time not pale yellowish dusty flatness like the Nullarbor, but deep reddish-coloured terrain with outcrops of rockiness. Very soon I was to clamber among these types of rocks with a tray of medicines in my hand doing my lunchtime medication round for a small tribe of Aboriginal inpatients. I already sensed the uniqueness of my forthcoming task.

After landing and travelling by car from the airstrip to the hospital, the doctor and pilot left me to go and do their weekly clinic. That old loneliness welled up in me again. I must be mad, I thought to myself, but there was no turning back now.

I unpacked my things into the room allotted to me in the nurses' home. As mentioned, Laverton Hospital was not a B.C.A. post, but a hospital owned and run by the Western Australian Government, so the place looked much as I would expect if it were a small country hospital anywhere. The home housed nurse assistants as well, a group of very committed but untrained personnel employed out of necessity to care for patients. Getting Registered Nurses to work in these out of the way towns was very difficult, and the present Matron had been the only RN for some time until joined recently by a nurse sent out from the W.A. Emergency Nursing Service. At the same time as I was arriving in Laverton, another two B.C.A. nurses were going to Derby in the northwest of Australia. My co-worker Helen was to join me in about a month, having first to finish off a nurse teaching position in Sydney.

Unpacking completed I came out of the nurses home door to be confronted with a large group of Aboriginals trying to sell their artefacts. I honestly didn't know what to do, so somehow I managed to walk through the group, I think without upsetting anyone, and made my way across to the hospital to meet my new boss. What I found when I came across her I immediately liked. A large jovial lady with a big booming voice welcomed me. Brought up in India of British parents here was a truly unique human being. Jet black hair pulled up into a tight bun on top of her head. A somewhat sallow complexion pierced by a pair of penetratingly laughing black eyes, which I later found could become quiet fierce when provoked. Her husband, Laurie, who acted as hospital maintenance man, was different again. Definitely Australian, this man exuded sun-tanned, well-built, Aussie charm via a bright white-toothed smile and deep smooth voice. He befriended me immediately with a natural warmth and brotherliness, while his wife was at first, a little more circumspect. They had one child only a small boy named Alec. Still in shock mode, I don't think I asked her what I should do about buying artefacts, but just decided to work this out for myself next time I was faced with the problem.

The next day I was into the nursing work with a vengeance. The other Registered Nurse had been given a well earned day off, and

I was to work for the next month without a break to help with the workload. I looked forward to when Helen would arrive. A fellow Christian with similar views and aspirations was what I craved in this very new and totally strange environment.

My first shift was different to say the least. First there were two elderly Aboriginal ladies sitting in the treatment room waiting for some help, but I couldn't understand a word they were saying. I ran for Matron who laughed raucously and proceeded to communicate with them in a kind of stilted Wongi language. Key words here and there seemed to get her quite a long way, and I realised that I would have to make an effort to learn some of this language. The Wongi was the local Aboriginal tribe of the Laverton area, and they were still very tribal in their outlook and behaviour. The realisation came to me with electric force, that we the white man had spoilt their way of life with our refined sugars, easy shopping, and worst of all our 'grog'.

After finally dealing successfully with the two old ladies, it was time to do the treatments for the children. What I saw that first day horrified me completely. Here were these lovely little Aboriginal kids, and most of them had big holes in their eardrums due to recurrent ear infections. They also were continually beset with body sores, boils, and chest infections, which were not only a problem to them physically, but meant lots of time off school and therefore quite damaging disruption to their education. I dressed all their wounds and gave out their medicines, and then went to see the adult wards.

The floors had not been washed for some time, as the domestic staff had not turned up for work. Matron and Laurie had tried to employ as many Aboriginal workers as possible to give them a start, but their commitment to work was quite different from ours. More about this later. The floor was filthy, so I got out the mop, forgetting my hatred of housework, and mopped it as best I could.

The hospital was made up of two long adult wards, one for males and the other for females. The adult patients were almost exclusively Aboriginal women, some with new babies of which we delivered approximately one per month. Sometimes, white Australian mining accident victims stayed in the male ward, but this was quite rare. The bulk of the patients were the Aboriginal children, who slept in the children's ward, and when not needed for their treatments, during the day, generally played outside amongst the rocks. As well as these, there were a small number of babies in cots, whom we also took outside as much as we could.

All the Aboriginal children were delightful, and enveloped you with love, probably a legacy of the family-oriented way of life they were used to amongst their own people. The babies were breast-fed anything up to four or five years of age, and children went everywhere with their mothers. This of course, was a problem when you separated them on admission to hospital. The mothers could stay if they wanted to, and visit any time, but usually they had things to do, other children, and places to go, which meant that they could not be there all the time. These babes cried incessantly when left, and required very frequent feeding from a cup. Matron absolutely outlawed bottles. "They can't use them on the reserve", she explained. "So it is not safe for us to introduce them when in hospital." I admired her for that, but still found it difficult to keep these little ones happy on frequent swigs from a feeding mug or cup and spoon.

After work the first day I was sitting on my bed in my room in the nurse's home, door wide open and other female workers visiting, when one of the male members of the hospital staff arrived in the doorway without so much as a knock. I was astonished at his apparent feeling of freedom to infiltrate our female living quarters so blithely. We were discussing what we would do that evening, with him sitting uninvited on the bed beside me listening in, when I said I would probably join the others in the usual trip to the local pub. Immediately he moved up the bed closer to me, the respect I had felt from him on my arrival seemed to have dissipated instantly. My thought processes went into rapid reappraisal of my circumstances, and I decided there and then, that even if it were only for the opinion of me as a Christian by that man alone, I would never set foot in the Laverton Hotel, and I never did.

Back on the job again the next day, the other thing that hit me was infection control, or was it lack of infection control? My stint at the Royal Children's Hospital in Melbourne haunted me constantly. Put all the babies in the one bath together…never! But do it I soon did. Not only were they used to this togetherness, but with so many little people to look after and so few staff to do it, I had to succumb. Making up a cot I looked across at three little black babies sitting up in the bath and thought to myself, "If only they could see me at home now, they would be horrified." But I still had a giggle. They looked gorgeous. The other pastime I was quickly initiated into was the ride in the clean linen trolley. On at least a daily basis we would pile all the littlies in the trolley and wheel them around the hospital grounds. After this all the clean hospital linen would go into this trolley. It was certainly a riot.

The days of my first month sped by, and still struggling with the culture shock, I suddenly realised it was time to go and get Helen.

CHAPTER 11 THE BISHOP, LINDA, AND MILES

When Helen was due, it was decided that we would meet in Kalgoorlie at the Bishop's residence. It is high time that Bishop Bryant should come into this story, because he and Linda (his wife) were definitely part of the whole romance of this outback experience.

I had already stayed at their home on my way through to Laverton initially, and had been overcome by the love exuding from them both. On top of this they had stamped their unique style on to the home in which they lived, and one could not fail to be impressed by this. The Bishop was, among many other talents, an artist, and had painted small plaques for some of the doors inside the house. One guestroom had "some friends sleep here", the next "other friends sleep here", and his own bedroom a monk lying down with the caption "the Bishop and Lin. sleep here"! The bathroom of course had a plaque also, with a little monk standing in front of three taps: one marked hot, the next cold, and the third holy! The Bishop and his wife both laboured day and night in their God-given roles with the energy of teenagers, and they must have been at least 60. I loved them, not only for their constant caring, but also because of their conversion experience.

The Bishop had told me all about it one day when we were driving around Kalgoorlie. He had been a committed member of the Airforce when he decided to enter a church. He was almost immediately converted, but instead of going straight home to tell

Linda he decided to wait until she voluntarily joined him in his commitment without any instigation from him. He subsequently waited for eight months, continuing his work as if nothing had happened. I asked Mrs Bryant if she had noticed anything different about him during this time and she did say that he had seemed a little more distant from her than previously, and went for more walks on his own than he ever had before. They had been together ever since their teens, so she really had known him a long time. Then one night they had a few friends over and she decided to cook some bacon and eggs for supper. Linda had the bacon and eggs in the frying pan in her hand when she suddenly dropped it down in the kitchen and said to her husband: "I think you should become a minister." At this he broke down and cried, saying how long he had waited for that very moment. From then on they served their Lord together, but never ceased to infiltrate this service with their own inimitable styles. Many a time Linda could have been caught eating cheese and drinking beer in the kitchen of the Bishop's residence, (she usually hid it under the bench if anyone came to the door), not to mention her smoking habit, which she had tried unsuccessfully to overcome. I found these little weaknesses only helped one feel at home with her and her wonderful humanness. Anyway it was with them that Helen and I would start our acquaintance.

" I got you a ride to Kalgoorlie to pick up Helen." Laurie looked pleased with himself as he recounted the tale. He had been down to the local hotel to find a travelling salesman friend of his, and called to him through the bathroom door. "How would you like to give a ride to a lady to Kalgoorlie?" "How old is she?" the guy immediately replied. "About 25," said Laurie. "I'll take her," he said. I asked the salesman later if he would have taken me if I had been an old lady. "No way" he immediately answered.

Miles was a cheerful-looking Aussie bloke, and turned out to be as friendly as he looked. The trip which normally took about four hours, went on all day, because Miles had to call in at all his selling contact points along the way and spend time with customers. He was a pleasant travelling companion, and I enjoyed his conversation. Having missed out on the Laverton pub, I made up for it with visits to all the 'watering houses' on the southbound road. With me it was always inevitable that we talked about religion. I really couldn't help it because from my point of view it pervaded every aspect of life. Miles was a little nonplussed. "Meditate a bit for me", he said when he left me in the car at one stopover.

We chatted along the rest of the way and I had enjoyed the trip, but it was still a surprise to me on reaching Kalgoorlie, that he asked if I would like to go out with him. Due to a feeling of commitment to the reason for which I was in Kalgoorlie in the first place, I declined, and in later lonely months in Laverton I was sorry that I had not made a friend of him. I always hoped afterwards that he might drop in on one of his many trips through the region, but I never saw him again. That encounter was to be but the first of many such meetings with unattached young men throughout my sojourn. I realised that one big problem with the outback was the unavailability of eligible females. My inbuilt stipulation of requiring a committed Christian for a partner, and my determination to remain a virgin at all costs until I found the person of God's choice for me, if ever I found such a one who was also compatible that is, probably saved me from many an alliance which may not have been in the best interests of either me or my calling. That's not to say I wasn't sad though as I let each attractive male opportunity pass me by.

Miles dropped me outside the Bishops residence in Kalgoorlie in the darkness of early evening, and Linda Bryant welcomed me with open arms at the door.

CHAPTER 12 HELEN AND I

Helen was a dark-haired attractive girl, with lots of bounce and fun in her. She had recently been teaching final year nursing students so I knew that she must be clever. As she was to be my co-worker for approximately two years, I was a bit nervous about meeting her, but as I renewed my already happy relationship with the Bryant's and Helen was introduced, I relaxed, and we all sat down to talk. It was only then that I realised just how traumatic my first three months with B.C.A. had really been. I relived the first two months relieving and then the month at Laverton, as the other three listened with sympathy. I'm not sure if my honesty was all that helpful for Helen who was yet to become enmeshed, but in those days I was always a little selfish about my own problems, and usually sought some outlet for sharing with those around me should they be willing to listen. Here was a captive audience, and in the warmth of that atmosphere I practically talked myself out. We went to bed quite late and I slept heavily. I was not looking forward to going back.

Helen and I returned to Laverton the next day with the Flying Doctor Service as I had done before. Helen's first evening on duty we worked alone together and she saw some of the difficulties I had tried to describe in Kalgoorlie. Towards the end of the shift we were giving out the medications. All the Aboriginal children patients usually chose to sleep two to a bed, and none of them ever had nametags. We were desperately trying to discover which child was which until finally we had to resort to pulling down one child's pants to see if it was a boy or a girl! We laughed about this many times after and relieved a bit of our stress. Following this first night we never worked together again, as R.N.s were scarce and we only used one to a shift.

It wasn't long before some of the real problems became apparent, and I realised that life in Laverton was not going to be pleasant in every circumstance. Some people drank very heavily every night at the pub and one night after one of these bouts one of the townspeople arrived up at the hospital where I was on duty alone. I was not expecting any nastiness from this hitherto charming man, so was horrified when he sat me down on a bench on the verandah and defying my continued requests to be released to continue caring for my patients, forced me to listen to a tirade of incoherent and endless discourses. For much of the time he spent there, and it must have been at least an hour, I could not understand what he was on about, until finally he ended up with what for me was a chilling statement. "Do not" he said, "bring church into this hospital". As he spoke these words he glared at me menacingly, and I was acutely conscious of his immense physical strength. Following that final enlightening statement, he went home.

I was quite shaken after that incident and not quite sure where to go from there. Helen and I had not yet sorted out just what form our Christian outreach in Laverton might take, and we both agreed that this new development was not going to be very helpful. We discovered that there was an evangelical Christian family living on the way to town, and we went there to visit them. They were running services regularly and I decided to attend when work permitted. The fellowship was good but so little in a place so barren, especially from a religious point of view. One of the B.C.A. ministers from Boulder W.A. came at intervals also, but in between we remained mostly alone with our philosophy.

The other problems were also difficult to handle. The Aboriginal health situation already mentioned seemed to us to be unresolvable. The children recurrently hospitalised for the aforementioned sores, ear, and chest infections, were also nearly always infested with scabies and lice. No one ever suggested repairing their severely ruptured eardrums either, and addressing these problems seemed to be an insurmountable obstacle. Most of Laverton's Aboriginal population lived on the reserve at the edge of the town, and quite near to the hospital. By law we were not permitted to go onto the Reserve, as these areas were supposed to provide privacy and protection for the inhabitants. The trouble was that tribal Aboriginals were not used to living in any kind of house, and the accommodation built for them seemed inappropriate. When one of my patients took off home one day before his treatment was finished, I was forced to follow to bring him back. It was then that the full impact of his lifestyle became clear to me.

The shell-like houses they lived in were dilapidated and dirty. I would hope they had been built with the best of intentions, but the inhabitants obviously had no understanding of how to utilise this kind of house. They also slept with their dogs, which looked half-starved to me, and used their meagre welfare payments to buy very low quality foods from the shops in town. As I peered in at the state of my patient's home, I understood more of the reason for the recurrent illnesses which seemed to beset some of the families, and felt sad that, at that time anyway, there seemed to be little we could legally do to alter this. Much later, just before we left Laverton, the Government finally employed a public health nurse who was allowed onto the reserve, and this was the start of the eventual improvement of the whole situation some years afterwards.

As in Coober Pedy, the Flying Doctor visited once a week. In between we managed somehow to deal with all that came our way. One day I was concerned at the squeaky cry of a new Aboriginal baby, as a squeaky cry could mean increased intracranial pressure, possibly due to a meningitis infection or a brain haemorrhage. As it was Doctors day I asked the doctor to have a look at this child. He could find nothing wrong, and I had to admit that Aboriginal babies often had somewhat squeaky cries under normal circumstances. Later that afternoon, the Doctor long gone, I returned to the mother's bedside to check out this babe. To my horror I noted a bulging fontanelle, fontanelle being the medical name for the small area on top of a baby's head where the skull bones have not yet united. The skull bones are like that at birth, so that they can overlap to give a smaller diameter during the birthing process—this area usually closes over completely by about eighteen months of age. This bulging was the classic sign in an infant, of an already too late to treat bacterial meningitis. The babe died very soon afterwards and I have never forgotten the trauma of this incident. The facts are that one almost has to treat this problem with the appropriate antibiotics before the signs and symptoms are clearly manifested, to prevent brain damage, and how I wished we had just decided to treat it in case earlier in the day. Many years later as a nurse educator I taught infectious diseases to third year nurses, and always shared this story with them to try to create an awareness of the problem.

It was Matron's idea that all sick Aboriginal children should be admitted, as she felt that their parents would be unable to care for them satisfactorily. In Coober Pedy we had sent them home with simple instructions and mostly they had seemed to cope quite well, but as mentioned previously, Laverton's native people were still quite tribal, so they may not have managed. It was nothing to go looking for inpatients to give them medicines, and find them sitting beside a newly-lit camp-fire chewing Kangaroo bones and chatting away in their colourful language. That language was still a difficulty. We needed to understand more to be able to help them properly, so we set about learning as much of it as we could.

In this new world suturing was also part of our daily routine. My first one was a simple cut on an Aboriginal lady's arm, and after coping quite well with that, I felt ready for anything except for what came next. A white chap who had been in a car accident arrived at the clinic. With blood all over his face and no obvious cuts, I lifted up his heavy black hair which fell naturally low down on his forehead. To my dismay his scalp came too, at least to halfway along the top of his head, so I dropped the hair down again and considered my options. I had hitherto never dealt with anything like this, but I knew there was no-one around to help, so I got organised and went on and sewed up the head on my own. Shortly after, one of the policemen in town came in, and seeing my handiwork, complimented me on it. After that I felt I could handle anything, medical that is, and over the rest of the three years with B.C.A. I just about had to.

But the spiritual side of things did not improve. Helen and I prayed about this together but found few direct answers. We made friends with the townspeople but were unable to commence any organised Christian outreach. I started helping a nurse assistant with an alcohol problem, and in my loneliness, became very dependent on her friendship. This was a situation which never became morally wrong, but I felt it was not helpful either, so, much later, when I had already left Laverton, I broke contact with her in order that each of us would learn to function with only God as our support. I still believe, no matter how we are tempted otherwise, that this is the right way to be, even in a marriage. Helen and I both did our best to help and care for everyone we met, but nevertheless, we grieved badly over our seeming failure to fulfil our calling to formally bring the love of Christ to this place.

The Aboriginal people were very keen to talk about God and to assimilate Him into their own religion, but the white people of the town were openly hostile, even to the point where one of the policemen sarcastically suggested to me that I should really be a nun not a nurse if I was wanting to tell anyone else about the faith. What also seemed to make things worse, was that one of the other policemen decided to have a crush on me. He constantly visited the hospital to seek me out, giving people golden opportunities to make crude public remarks about what he may or may not have had in his mind about me. He never made any untoward advances, but the inferences were always lurking.

I must admit though that in the midst of these traumas, we did have some good times. There was the local Laverton Hospital Ball which Helen attended. People came from as far away as Perth—so friendly and inviting us to visit them in their homes if we ever came South. That was one thing about W.A., apart from those who were hostile to Christianity, the people were often most hospitable.

The football team was likewise a real hit. The nearest town south from us was Leonora, also a mining town, and similarly small and barren. They were the only available competitors for footy, so one week Laverton would play Leonora, the next Leonora would play Laverton, and so on until for the final, Laverton would play Leonora! With the incredible lack of rain the ground would be a dust bowl where one could hardly distinguish the players, and when they came off the field at the end of a match, they generally looked just like pillars of dirt.

Then there was the time we were told that Brian Viney was coming to see us. Helen and I looked at one another. "Who's Brian Viney?" we said. Afterwards we felt ashamed. He was only the current W.A. Secretary for the Bush Church Aid Society!

When Brian arrived we both liked him instantly. Here was a warm, engaging man, sympathetic to our problems, but also a great tease. We enjoyed his visit and on his departure Helen said to me: "You've got four days off Audrey, why not drive down with Brian and visit Perth." What a great idea! I was packed in an instant and off we went.

Seventy miles down the road as we entered Leonora, I said to Brian. "I had better phone back and let Matron know where I am." A handy phone box presented itself and Laurie answered the phone. "Where are you," he shouted. "Going to Perth with Brian" I answered. "B— H—" he exclaimed, "You've only just met him." Laurie had no idea of the immediate rapport and trust which can exist between like-minded Christians. Brian and I had a good chuckle about that.

The trip was a great time of fellowship, as was the time spent in Perth with Brian's wife Margaret and their children. It was a veritable oasis in the midst of the spiritual drought in which Helen and I were enmeshed. I confided to Brian that I didn't know when to buy the Aboriginal artefacts which the Laverton locals constantly begged us to purchase. "When you want them," he said gently. Why hadn't I thought of such a simple and fair answer to a problem? Brian and his family had brought a touch of healing to my sagging spirits. I took a plane back to Laverton on a blue, blue sky day, and took up the reins again.

CHAPTER 13 STAFFING THE HOSPITAL

One of the wonderful things about Matron and Laurie when they arrived in Laverton first, was their desire to employ as many of the local indigenous population as they could in the running of the hospital. They recounted their experiences in fulfilment of this objective with a degree of disappointment that their success was somewhat sparse, because when Helen and I arrived the total Aboriginal staff consisted of about three nurse assistants and one laundress. "What was the problem?" I asked Laurie. "Some days they just didn't turn up if they didn't feel like it," he said. "Can't run a hospital like that so we had to go back to non-Aboriginal workers." He sounded genuinely disillusioned but I felt that this couldn't be taken at face value, so I decided to reserve judgement on the issue. As the weeks and months ambled by I came to a conclusion. Aboriginal people were not lazy at all. When they worked they did a beautiful job, as good as or better than non-Aboriginal, but they did not seem to have any concept of guilt where work was concerned. I felt that some of the time, if not all of it, non-Aboriginal workers that I knew and had known, including myself, worked hard not only because we had to, but often because we would not like someone else to think that we were not pulling our weight, whereas my experience of Aboriginals so far, was that they did not have a problem with what other people thought of them. If they felt like working they would, if not they wouldn't, and I believe they expected their co-workers to behave in like manner. Then they would say, "What is the problem?" as long as someone is working. It was a totally different ballgame to them. I felt absolutely no animosity towards them while I was there, and they were, on the whole, very loving towards me. There was only one girl whom I felt exhibited what I called reverse racism towards me, and by this I mean that she seemed to expect that I would discriminate against her, and pre-empted what she thought I was going to do or say before I had a chance to move in any direction. I found this most unsettling because try as I might to tell her I wasn't feeling as she thought, she did not seem to want to believe me. We went on a few outings together which were spoilt by this problem.

Apart from this I met some truly beautiful Aboriginal people: the Matron of Leonora hospital, families in Laverton, other co-workers, and fellow Christians, especially at the nearby missions. Their faith was one of the most beautiful things about them. It was simple, glowing, warm, and disarmingly real. I truly loved them for that.

Nevertheless the staffing of the hospital seemed best accomplished by using people from a Perth agency, mostly young and on working holidays. What a great bunch of girls we met there, way out the back of nowhere, friendly, capable, adventurous…their company was life-saving, but Helen and I continued to struggle, until suddenly my mother summoned me home for a family crisis.

CHAPTER 14 THE FIRST ESCAPE

Getting away from the scene of a traumatic situation usually gives one space to reassess. What was wrong, what should be done, what was to blame if anything? My mother was always a listening ear, and often solutions would come when I poured out the problems to her. I helped resolve the family situation and then tried to sort out my own, but to no avail. I hadn't enjoyed the B.C.A. hospitals so I felt that I couldn't go back there, and besides I didn't think there were any vacancies in that direction yet. Somewhere along the line I heard that the girls at Derby were struggling too. I empathised. Could I leave the Society altogether? After all I could hardly be considered a blistering success! No spiritual work commenced, allowing myself to be traumatised by people's threats, and leaning on my new Laverton friend, more than was good for either of us. But, I saw no option, so I went back.

CHAPTER 15 UNCONTROLLABLE HEAT AND A COMMITMENT INCOMPLETE

Back across the Nullarbor I went and when I alighted from the train at Kalgoorlie it was like walking into a great big oven. The temperature was soaring and I loved it, but that didn't alter my sense of foreboding for lifting up again the burden of ministry in Laverton. My friend met me at the train, grateful that I had indeed returned because she thought I wouldn't. She had borrowed one of the Laverton policemen's cars as hers was quite poorly at present, and we set off on the long hard drive north. The roads were unmade in many parts, incredibly dusty and risky for windscreens, but that was not what went wrong. Water in the radiator ran dry, and by the time we reached Leonora, the head was cracked.

Policeman and nurses were the best of friends in the outback. They helped us and we helped them. Contrary to public opinion in many areas today, the police in all my outback experience were very kind to Aboriginals, and if ever there were any children left on the loose because parents were in gaol or drunk, the police would bring them to the hospital and we would look after them. Alcohol was a problem to non-Aboriginals as well of course, but the Aboriginal seemed to be particularly adversely affected by the brew, to the point that originally it was decided not to allow them to have it. It was while Helen and I were in Laverton that drinking rights for Aboriginals in the area came in, and the Police Chief was quite concerned for he believed this would not help them, at least in the early days of getting used to this new freedom. He was not wrong. Children previously well looked after and well fed by their parents were found searching through rubbish bins for food and admitting themselves to hospital because of hunger. We all agonised over this. Anyway back to Leonora!

Still 70 miles to go and steam pouring forth from the radiator, we were hot, thirsty, and hungry, when rescued by you know who—the local constabulary. They then took us, in the back of the cage would you believe, to one of the police officers' own homes, where we were allowed to stay the night, not I might add behind bars! Very cordial I thought.

Next morning we phoned Merv in Laverton. He should have been incredibly annoyed that we had wrecked his car, but Merv was a very easy-going guy, with a broad friendly grin and brotherly demeanour. "I'll come and get you", he said, and did precisely that.

When we got back to the hospital I found that even more traumas had developed in my absence. We sat down quietly together and Helen explained. Matron had decided that the usual casual habit we all had of visiting the hospital when we were off duty to chat to one another was from now on to be outlawed. She said that it was out of control and disruptive, and that people had taken advantage of privileges. I'm sure she had her reasons for this edict, but nevertheless for us it was quite shattering. Here we all were in this very arid and inhospitable place. Nowhere much to go, practically no entertainment except for the odd party, overwhelming Aboriginal medical health problems, and a sparse white social structure which was not often nurturing, and she wanted to close us off from our most reliable source of sanity. At this point however, we had no choice but to continue.

I guess Helen and I didn't really know that God was not using us, it just seemed that way at the time. Later on the person who had told me not to bring church into the hospital actually changed his tune completely and said that if we ever did start a Sunday school in Laverton he would send his son along. Quite a change from his original feelings.

Also, at times there were other things to chuckle over or battle with which seemed to lighten the load or make things more worthwhile. One of the working holiday girls from Perth was sent to work with the lady in the laundry, and at first couldn't understand how this lady managed to get through so much washing so quickly. Watching carefully one day she discovered the secret. The washing was put in beautifully with the required amount of soap, but when this cycle was complete no rinsing was even thought about, the washing simply spun and hung on the line to dry. The weather always being so sunny it was dry enough to bring in at night, whereupon all pegs would be removed while the washing fell to the dry red dusty ground. So much easier to collect up in armfuls and take inside, than painstakingly holding each item as pegs were released!

Then one day we were notified of a very ill child at Warburton Ranges some 200km further inland (and I thought Laverton was the end of the line). Helen was co-opted to go with Laurie in the car. I stayed back hoping all would go well. Many hours later they returned safely with this small four-year-old girl in an advanced state of starvation and dehydration. Putting an intravenous into a child of this age was a difficult procedure, and to waste time trying to fly her to Kalgoorlie may be too late, so we proceeded to feed her dry cereal mixed with tap water via a stomach tube inserted down her nose, a treatment we were all trained to cope with very well. We took it in turns overnight to feed her very small amounts frequently, and continued on throughout the ensuing days increasing the feeds as tolerated. After some weeks she became a plump healthy and adorable little person whom we all loved. Her name was Veronica, but for some reason we called her Veronipush, which seemed to suit her beautifully. What a success and a fulfilment.

We also delved into midwifery, an area which I really loved. One night when Helen was on Night Duty we decided to play a trick on her, as she was not so fond of the obstetric realm. Breaking the taboo re visiting the hospital, several of us climbed into hospital beds with pillows on our stomachs and our heads covered in blankets calling out "Bega, Bega lara" meaning sore, very sore in Wongi. At the handover Helen was horrified. One mid. was bad enough but three!! Her look of utter disgust when she pulled back the blankets to check her charges, showed that Helen was not very impressed, but it did take our mind off other things for a little and Helen duly forgave us.

Helen was very creative with the children, still not my strong point, so while I enjoyed delivering the babies, about one a month in Laverton, she enjoyed organising the kids. Sometimes when I came on duty, she would have all the children sitting on the mat in front of the open fire which was always lit when nights were cold, pretending to be in a boat rowing their way to shore. They loved this kind of role-play and Helen was very good at instigating this sort of activity.

I never ceased to be thrilled by the new little babies, and one of the funniest moments came when we took a new Aboriginal baby, born overnight, into the room where all the small inpatients were sitting on the floor in a circle waiting for their treatment. An Aboriginal assistant held up the babe and asked the children where they thought this exquisite bundle of joy came from. "New Guinea", was the immediate reply. We laughed so much it did us all the world of good.

Another treatment session ended similarly when we were chatting as we dressed the children's boils and sores. You know how we Australians will often brag about ourselves saying we are famous for our charm, personality, etc. etc. whereupon one of the Aboriginal nurse assistants added "and Specific Gravity"! We were absolutely endeared to her from then on.

Despite these lighter interludes, for both Helen and I the traumas persisted, and all finally came to a head with a visit from our W.A. administrator Stan Hummerston. Stan was a Godsend who listened to all our woes and made some wise decisions for us. It was with much sadness at our seeming failure, that Helen and I finally left Laverton after only eight months service there, she to return to Sydney where she eventually married, and me…well despite my previous misgivings, it was back to Cook!

In retrospect regarding Laverton, I now believe no time is wasted where God is concerned. We did not know whom we may have influenced, and we had helped staff that little Government Hospital all those months. But most of all we had grown, even though painfully, we were not the same Helen and Audrey who had entered that scene. We were now ready for God's next step.

LAVERTON W.A.

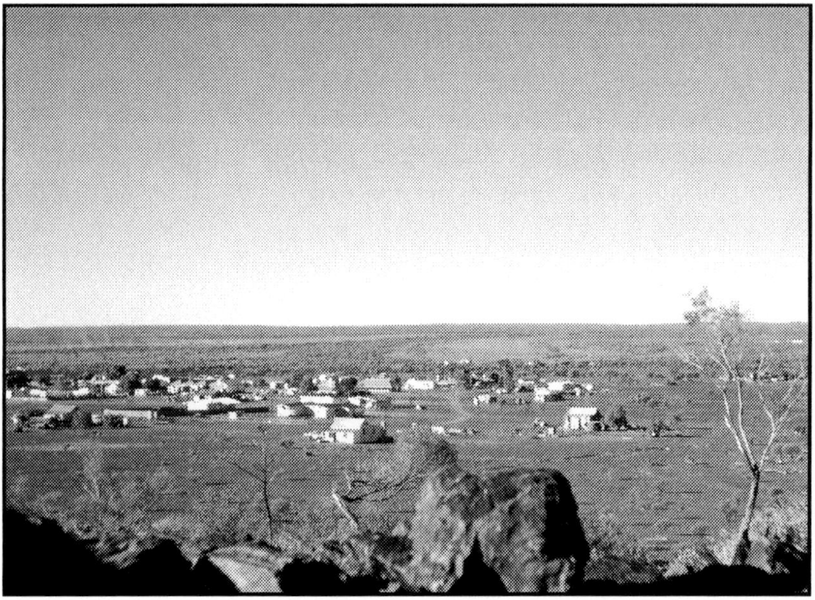

Laverton township, 1971

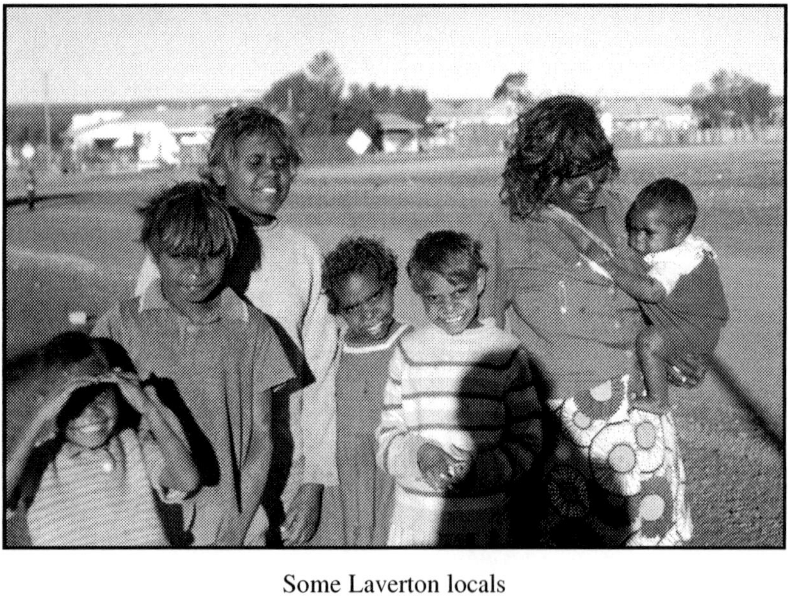

Some Laverton locals

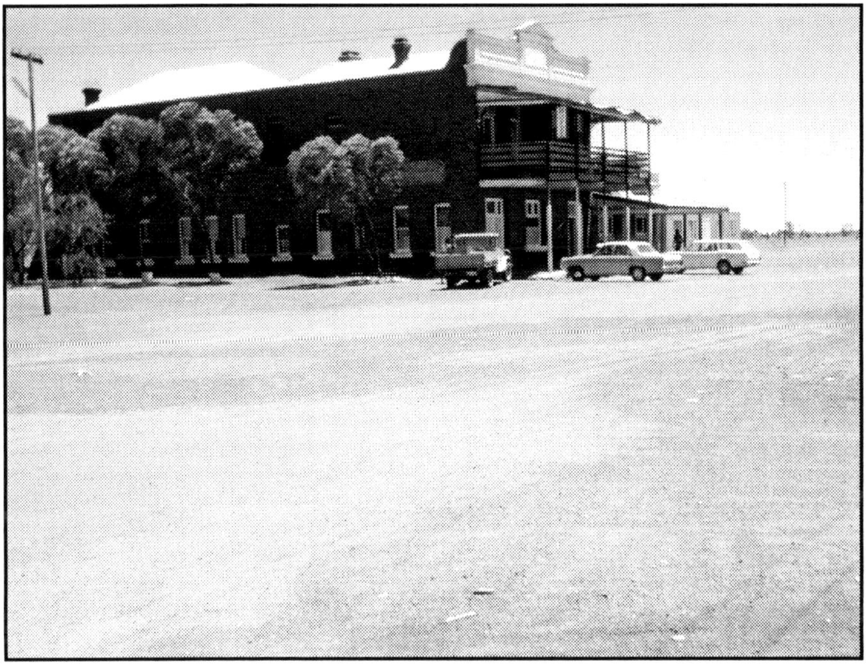

Laverton Hotel

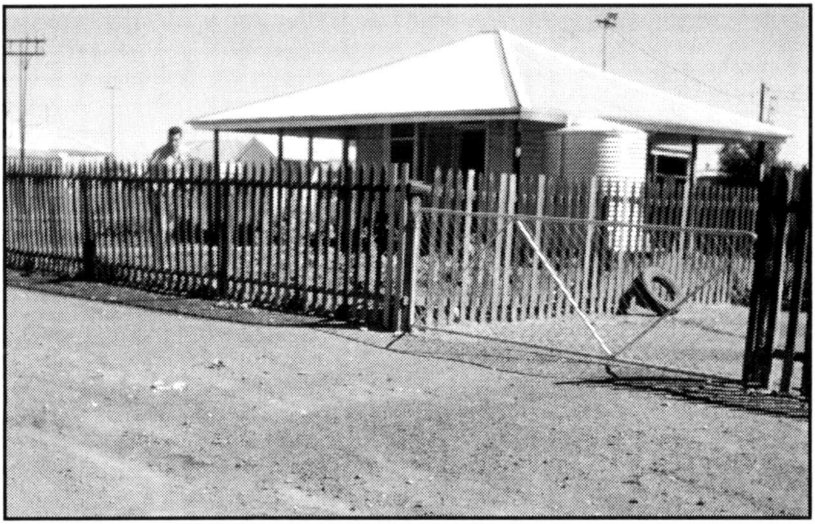

Laverton Police Station

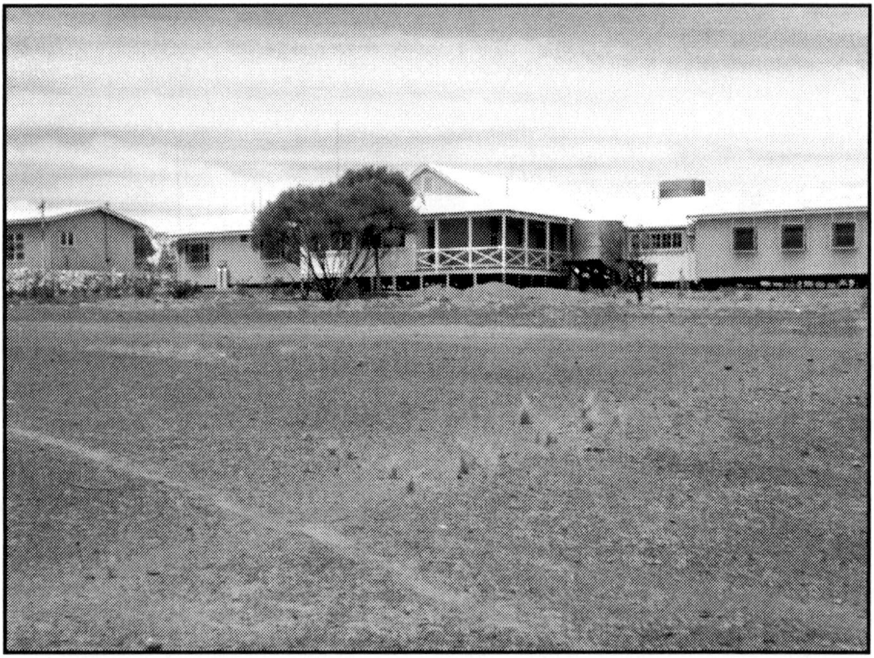

Laverton Hospital

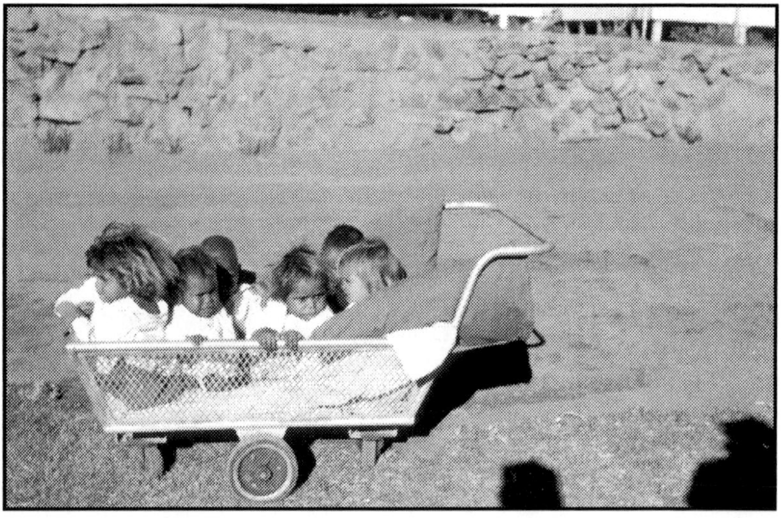

Little patients out for a walk—Laverton Hospital

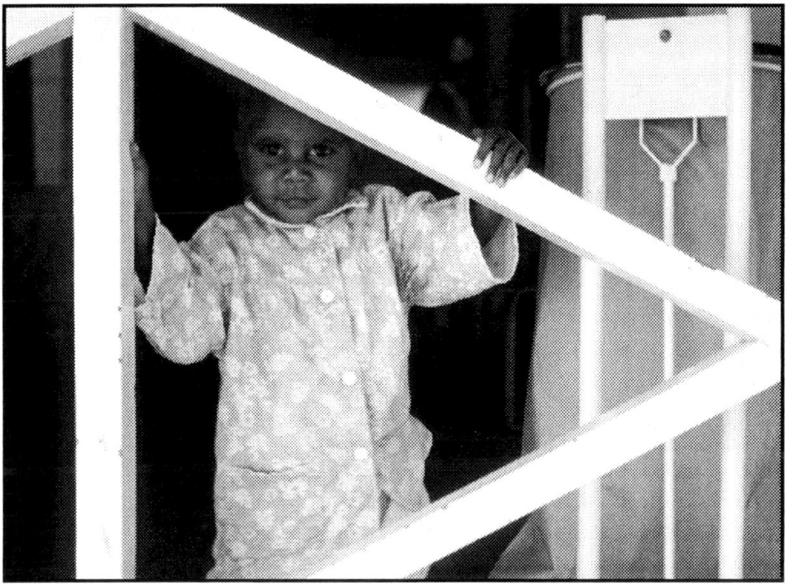

Veronica

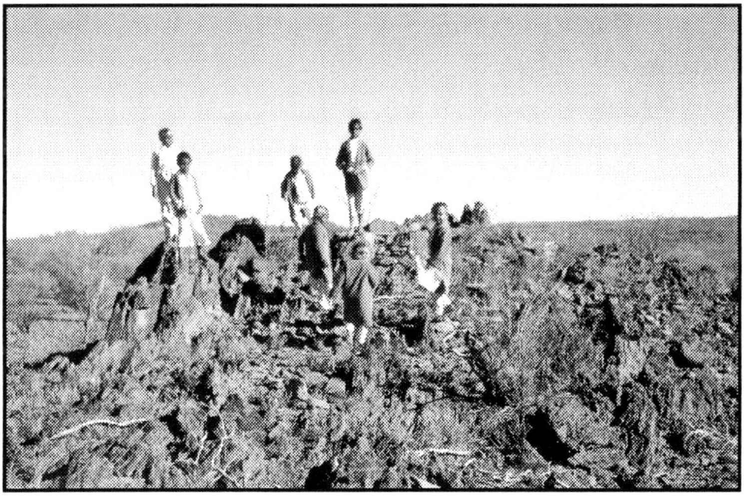

Young patients in Laverton Hospital grounds

CHAPTER 16 BACK TO COOK

It was amazing for me that the very place which I had left with relief only some ten months prior, I was now returning to with a distinct feeling of joyous anticipation. My only explanation was that this may have been what God had planned all along, but initially I was not ready for it. In His wisdom He knew that Laverton was not to be my place of ministry, just a place which would hone me for the task of His choice, and it had definitely done that. After Laverton I was happy to go just about anywhere! Added to this, Ruth had just finished up and returned to England, so there was the vacancy ready and waiting for me to just slip into. As usual, God's timing was perfect.

Carol was happy because she knew me from before, and felt that we would get on well together. Sometimes getting on together was a problem with which we found Christian workers had to battle quite hard, particularly when working in isolated places with people they had never met before. Pam and Brian were happy too because they had been praying for someone to come who would fit into the situation harmoniously. They sent me a telegram communicating their enthusiasm for my new appointment. I felt at peace.

My Laverton friend wanted to take me down to Kalgoorlie to catch the train. Her own car was now mobile so fortunately there was no need to borrow. She was devastated when I said I was going. For the past months of our friendship she had managed to control her alcoholism, but without me neither of us knew if she could continue to do so. As I have discussed already, I knew that no-one should be that dependant on another person, that God was really the best one to lean on so completely, but often we feel we are unable to manage with only Him. I think it is then that He removes the very people or things we are leaning on the most, to help us see that He really can fulfil all our needs. This girl was definitely a person of faith, and was about to be forced into a period of real spiritual growth. Nevertheless I was not happy being the one to cause this pain, and I therefore promised at this stage to keep in touch.

We spent a very sad day in Kalgoorlie, and then she took me to the train. My policeman friend was on the platform. He had driven, by the look of him, in some kind of frenzy, down from Laverton to see me before I left. He never said the things to me I believe were in his heart. He wasn't very good at communicating his feelings at the best of times, having often appeared at the hospital in Laverton with the obvious intention of seeing me yet always leaving without having made any definite move. When I was on duty the night of the Laverton ball he strode angrily into the kitchen where I was folding linen and demanded to know why I had to work when the ball was on, and then left without saying why it mattered to him. And here he was, tall and well built but looking lost and neglected. He kissed me and I said goodbye. I felt I had let him down but knew nothing could be done. I had other work to do. I could only pray that he would find his niche and be able to make some sense of life's many disappointments. I prayed for him for many years after and as yet have not heard of him again.

Memories of my first trip across the Nullarbor filtered through my mind as the train made its way from Kalgoorlie. I thought of my Laverton friends standing on the platform. It is always harder to be the ones left behind. I looked forward to Cook this time, and put Laverton and its traumas behind me. The familiar warmth of the Nullarbor lay ahead.

Sitting in the train I found myself chatting comfortably to a young farmer from W.A. Watch it, I said to myself, you're doing it again, and I wasn't wrong. When I left the train at Cook this nice man wanted to keep in touch and didn't seem to know how to take no for an answer. For a while afterwards he wrote to me and even came back through Cook a year later to renew the acquaintance, but as I knew this was another "Miles'" experience I had to decline. I still wonder what happened to him.

Alighting from the train at Cook this was a completely different feeling from the first time. Now I knew the people, my co-worker, the type of work, and the trauma from which I had come. Now began a truly rewarding task. Carol had been trained for ministry as well as nursing. With her strength and organisational skills behind all the moves, and because we got on so well together, without over-dependency, our spiritual lives prospered, and I for one was greatly fulfilled by it all. Besides this we actually had a lot of fun, running all the Christian activities that I had been orientated to on my first visit to Cook. This time I felt I was becoming proficient at these things, as well as learning all the time. This was really walking with God, who also would have known the eventual outcome of the definite spiritual seed sowing that was going on. More about this later.

Meanwhile I agonised over what to do about my friend in Laverton. I knew this was unfinished business, so for the first and only time in my life so far, I fasted and prayed, and knew clearly what I must do. I wrote to her and told her that I would no longer be communicating with her. I knew how she would be in that empty place, so I also wrote to the B.C.A. minister responsible for visits to the area. How nice to know one had someone like that to call upon. Some months later he replied. She had become inebriated for four months he said, the thing which I had most feared, but then she had broken free of her addiction to alcohol, and become a powerful witness for the Lord in Laverton. I praised and thanked Him, who knew already the outcome before the deed, and perhaps could only use her fully when she was free of me. At least that is how I hoped it was.

Routines at Cook became very comforting. Every morning after breakfast and cleaning duties we would hop into the V.W. much as I remembered from the first time, and drive down to town. Mail collected and greetings to everyone we met, we'd wander into the store for items needed. The store was much like those I remembered in country Victoria, as well as the prices which were usually quite steep. Many of the townspeople were virtually owned by the Railways and unable ever to move anywhere else due to financial constraints. Some however were enterprising enough to save their minuscule salaries and travel up the line to a larger and cheaper town and buy in bulk. Eventually this pattern repeated would lead to an ability to complete one's financial commitment to the Railways and move up in the world and off the transline, but for many this never became a reality.

As noted on my first visit to Cook, once a week on Saturday evenings was the trip to the Tea and Sugar train to buy our meat on the train which travelled up and down the line visiting all the settlements small and larger along the way. There was a railway staff settlement approximately every seventy miles, most of them only six houses in size. Six families with under school age children would live in simple wooden houses with not even a radio or other heating and cooking besides the ever-present wood stove. One of the girls who had lived there and moved to Cook when her children needed a school camp spoke of how she and her neighbour used to rush through their housework and then sit in the colder months with their feet in the wood stove oven to keep them warm while they chatted the hours away. I wondered how I would have coped. For many of them a trip up the line in the goods train to visit the hospital, which was always a free trip, was the only available outing!

The Transcontinental trains passed through Cook at 8 AM and 8 PM every day, and stayed for half an hour while they were refuelled and rewatered. One brightspark passenger was heard to say one day while he was merrily cleaning his teeth on the dirt platform, "I wonder what all these people are doing out here while he stared incredulously at all of us. I felt like sharply informing him that if it weren't for the likes of us he wouldn't be able to travel on the train, for our presence was vital to the well being of the trains, but I kept it to myself because I wasn't sure that he would understand. I must say though that the reassuring sound of the trains coming and going, including the daily goods trains, were a great comfort to us, and sorely missed whenever there was a strike. As well as this they regularly brought friends to see us.

Ron was a train driver who lived with his wife and family in Kalgoorlie, and regularly stayed overnight at Cook before taking the train back the next day. Ron always came to visit us especially I think because he was a committed Christian and saw our encouragement as part of his ministry. Ron was a great guy, another real tease plus a very down to earth bloke. He often shared humorous anecdotes with us not the least being the time one of his kids dropped a brick down the toilet and his wife didn't know what to do with the water pouring everywhere so she tried to get in touch with him. Did he ever get teased about that for many moons after, as the guy whose kid broke the dunny and his wife couldn't cope without him. Nevertheless he seemed to adore his wife and proudly told us more than once that despite his full figure his wife's waist was still as small as the day he married her which I imagined meant that it was somewhat enviably tiny.

The passenger trains also brought patients from time to time, who definitely had not planned to be clients of Bishop Kirkby Memorial Hospital. One lady was eight months pregnant and decided she wanted to have the baby in Kalgoorlie, so she illegally hopped on the train in her heavily gravid state only to come into good labour half-way across the Nullarbor. The conductor contacted us whereupon we removed the poor girl from the train and flew her back to Port Augusta from whence she had come. I felt very sorry for this lady thwarted in her belated attempts at a W.A. delivery.

Fortunately too, Cook was not all work and no play. As well as the battinton on Thursday nights, very rarely there was also a movie show in the local hall. I remember well seeing Animal Farm and being suitably horrified by it. Saturday nights at Pam and Brian's continued, and John the young 'schoolie' joined in as he was boarding with them. These more junior teachers were sent to Cook without any choice, and some of them found the isolation very difficult. Later when he was transferred to Coober Pedy and Carol and I were also there, we caught up with him again which was a pleasant reunion. As did we, he found Coober Pedy a much more stimulating post with a drive-in theatre, numerous clubs, and many more young people than Cook or Tarcoola.

Buying clothes was a fascinating situation from somewhere as isolated as Cook. We were heavily into mail ordering and I eventually joined the others in both this and making my own clothes! I had some years previously done a formal course in dressmaking but had never been very successful at it. Now I started, with Carol's help making clothes in earnest and even finding them wearable. Amazing! Never having had much time at home to knit either, I could redevelop this previously quite well understood skill and happily knitted at every opportunity as did most of the women of Cook—much to the disgust of John who was sick of clicking knitting needles at every turn!

One chore I still didn't enjoy much was those monthly meetings of the hospital auxiliary, but somehow I managed to assist by simply doing the best I could.

The medical ministry was quite varied and also included infant welfare and midwifery. As mentioned, I had studied both of these areas, and was quite happy to practise these specialties. Carol and I were privileged to deliver Pam's second baby boy at Cook hospital, and also to, a little later, become his godparents. What a thrill.

Back to the spiritual seed sowing. We did a lot of spiritual things, Carol and I together, but I wasn't sure how successful we were in our outreach until I personally experienced a number of what I would class as moments when God definitely showed himself to be clearly at work. Pam and Brian always shared

Sunday services with us and then, when we least expected it, along came Pam and Ray Bateman, another couple who joined us after being in Cook for quite a while. Katy and Paul were Catholics and also decided to participate. We started a daytime Bible Study where others of the local women came along, and all the other activities continued to be well patronised especially where the children were concerned and guess what—I grew to love and manage those children as I had never dreamt I ever would!

One day the children we taught at the Monday night club for so long were challenged by a visiting Christian teacher to accept Christ as their Lord, whereupon a number of them did, and the joy of their commitment truly shone out of their faces. I felt that without all the prior preparation, and years of Christian witness in that place by B.C.A. nurses, they would not have so easily understood and accepted such a step.

Other answers to prayer were also quite clear to me. Later when Carol had left Cook, and I was supposedly in charge, I decided to sell a two burner heater, thinking we did not need it. Some time after, I remembered that this very heater was sorely needed for winter doctor's days for the clinic room. Oh dear, it was still warm at present but what was I going to do in winter? So I prayed and shortly afterwards the person to whom I had sold the heater came up to me with the following words. "Audrey do you know anyone who would want that heater I bought from you because we are moving up north and will no longer need it". Can you imagine my relief, and she happily gave it back to me for nothing.

Finally, there was the time I was going home to Melbourne and I needed to take the air-conditioning motor to Adelaide for repair. At Cook station all the people helped me with various bundles etc. and settled me nicely on to the train, but as I travelled along I wondered how I was going to carry everything when we changed trains at Port Pirie, and when I walked down to my Uncle who would be waiting at the end of the platform when I arrived in Adelaide. Meanwhile while I was praying about this and expecting some cool guy to appear as a knight in shining armour and carry it for me, we stopped at a small station and I got out of the train asking other people in the carriage if they wanted anything from the kiosk. A little old lady with a bad leg thanked me kindly and requested a drink, so I bought her one, not ever dreaming that making her acquaintance would be of any possible use to me with my heavy motor carrying problem, but so much for my understanding of the workings of God. When we reached our destination my invalid companion procured a luggage trolley for herself, ordered that my luggage be put on her trolley, which she then very ably propelled along, leaving me perfectly free to carry the motor alone which was an equally possible feat for me. What a God.

I think I could have gone on at Cook with Carol forever, but unfortunately this is rarely allowed. Life deals out its good and bad times, and the pattern can be difficult to understand, especially at the time. After 12 months of wonderful service together, Carol decided it was time for her to move on to Coober Pedy, as she had already been at Cook some five years. I had learnt a lot from her and knew I would miss her, but believing that it was not yet my time to move, I elected to stay on and work with whoever came along next. Besides, going to Coober Pedy was not my idea of fulfilment. I had already been there and not exactly enjoyed myself. I also still had a fear that even though I could now cope with Cook, Coober Pedy, with all its busy Medical work, would always be way beyond my capabilities. Once again I was not aware of just how much I was underestimating God's enabling power.

CHAPTER 17 THE NEW PARTNERSHIP

My heart sank as my new co-worker stepped from the train. I knew as soon as I saw her that we were not going to get on. Why I felt this so early I have no idea. I resolved nevertheless to make a good go of it.

After Carol left, we tried to settle into a routine. Carol and I had had one which seemed to suit us both, but this was not to be with my new colleague. Everything I wanted she didn't, and vice versa. Each morning I prayed as usual, hoping for greater harmony, only to find the day dissolving into one disaster of disharmony followed by another. I began to understand incompatible marriages, and we hadn't even chosen one another.

To make things worse I suddenly developed a succession of very painful boils, just getting rid of one to be blessed with another. All this was probably a legacy of my Laverton days, but I could have done without it, especially at this time. Eventually I treated myself with antibiotics and cured the horrible things, and fortunately have never had one since.

Later I realised I had probably been far too rigid with this second working relationship at Cook, wanting to stick to my old routines with which I felt comfortable, and not considering that someone else might find them a problem. This aside though, I wondered if whatever I had done may have been destined not to work. Many times throughout my Christian life I have pondered these things. I know prayer can change relationships miraculously, because I had already experienced this. When a new Christian in

Sydney, I had spent the morning working in the infectious babies' nursery under a Staff Midwife who continually verbally maligned and mistrusted me. At lunchtime I was sitting alone on my bed in the nurses home with my door open and tears in my eyes, when an older Christian nurse walked by. Noticing my grief she stopped to ask what was the matter. I told her of my dilemma whereupon she immediately suggested that we should pray for my abuser. "Pray for her!" I burst out, "That is the last thing I want to do." Nevertheless I gave in and we sat together to ask God to help. I went back to the nursery and the Staff Midwife was niceness personified. I had received proof of the value of one of the most important messages of the gospel. "Pray for your enemies..." Many times since then I have experienced the same answers, but sometimes nothing happens. My belief now is that when prayer does not change things, one must look at what else one could be doing. I wanted to stay at Cook, and my new co-worker didn't seem to care about it, yet it was I who eventually had to go to save my sanity, and she was allowed to stay. When I finally gave in to this and moved to Coober Pedy, the peace I had lost in those painful six months flooded back in, and I knew that nothing short of the pressure I had been under would have forced me to leave Cook. God allowed my discomfort to continue until I obeyed him. Other times I do believe that one must sit it out, and the guidance for that comes when one tries to move out but there is nowhere to go. In this instance under discussion, one of the girls at Coober Pedy willingly agreed to move to Cook. She felt happy about it and I, though traumatised, eventually realised that this was right.

My incompatible co-worker was annoyed when I told her that I was going to Coober Pedy. "You must have told them (meaning the bosses in Melbourne and Sydney) that we weren't getting on" she accused me angrily. "I had to" I said sadly. "I couldn't take it any more." Throughout the time of our difficulties I had allowed our usual stream of caring visitors to come and go, longing to ask them for help but respecting my colleague's wish that we remain silent about our differences, until I wondered how low one could allow oneself to feel before one would completely fall apart. My mother had called me home again to help her with the sale of her father's much loved house, and I had gone and poured out all the trauma. We had sat in the kitchen and Mum had simply said: "What about Coober Pedy?" and despite the fact that as mentioned, I had always previously felt completely inadequate for that task, I experienced an instant calm about it. So I had done it. Rung the boss and made arrangements for the transfer. When I returned to Cook the wheels were already in motion, and I could not reverse them.

Nevertheless the devil had a field day with me that last month in Cook. The children accused me of disliking the people of Cook. I couldn't tell them the real reason for my leaving, and they never understood. There was also the fact that I loved Cook, but I was forced by my own inability to cope with the situation to leave it all behind. My throat was so taut for weeks, and even while I stayed a day or so with the flying Doctor and his wife in Port Augusta, the stress levels did not fall. The peace only came again when the plane flew over Coober Pedy, and I knew that I had done the right thing.

COOK S.A.

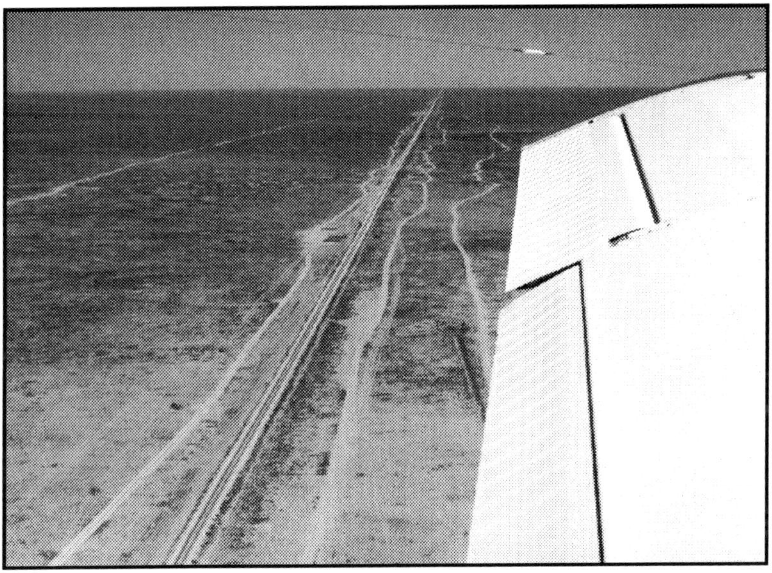

Aerial view of the Transline. S.A., 1972

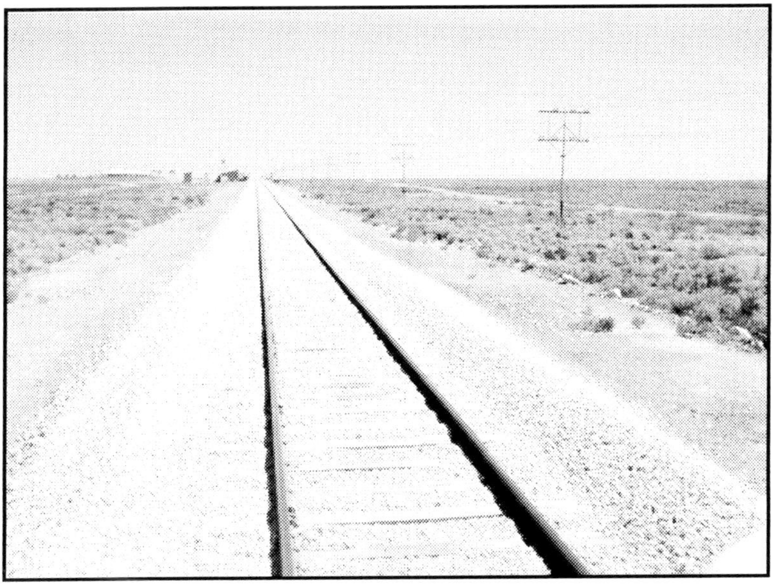

The Transline from the ground

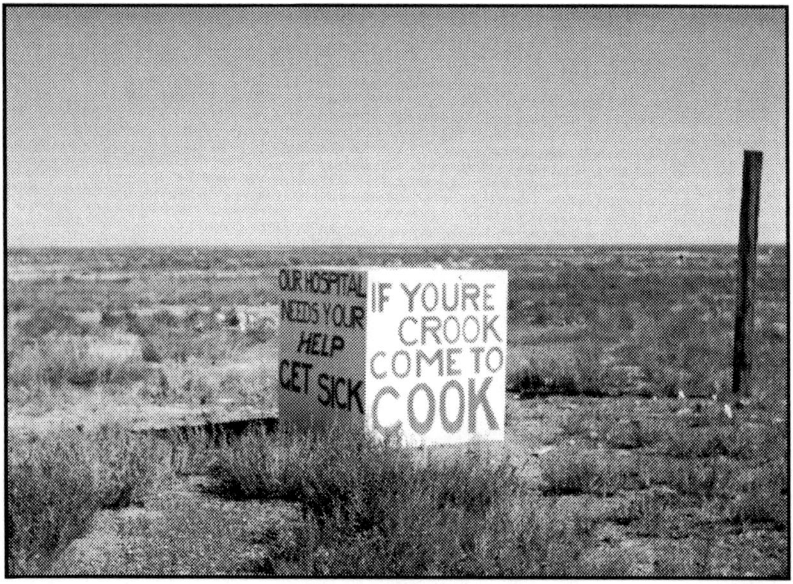

Plea to passengers

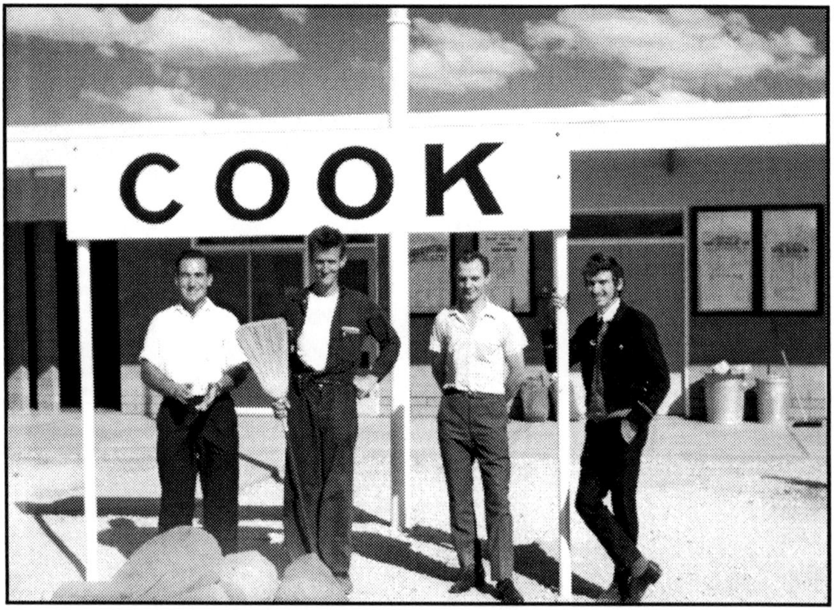

Railway workers at Cook Railway Station

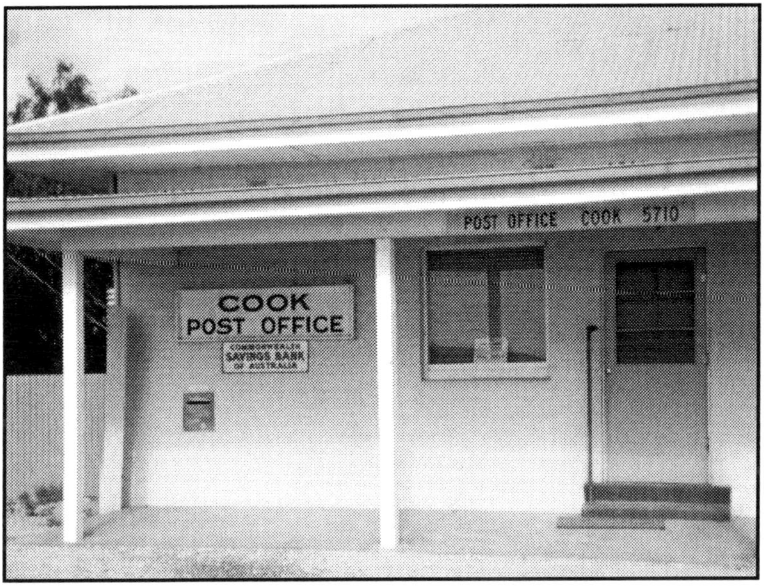

Cook Post Office

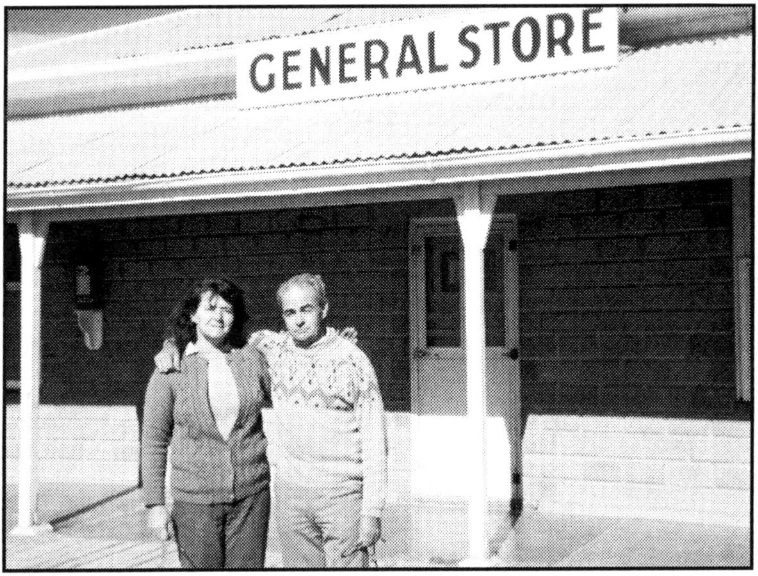

Cook General Store

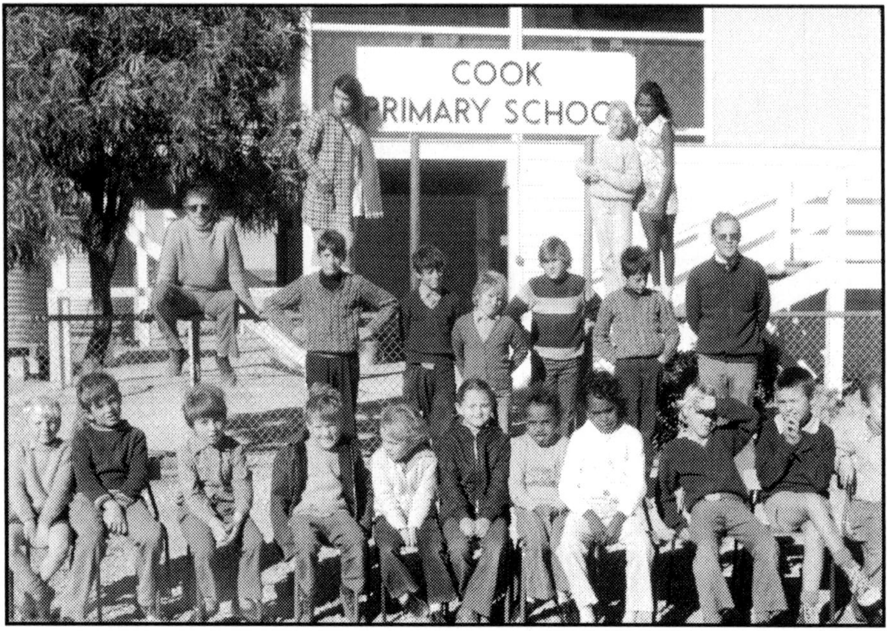

Cook Primary School

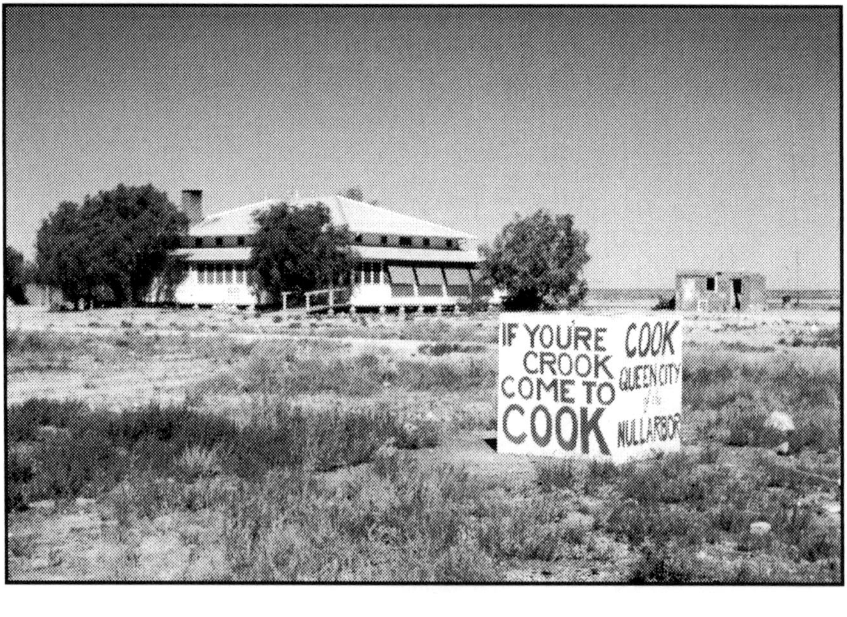

Cook Hospital with plea to passengers in the foreground

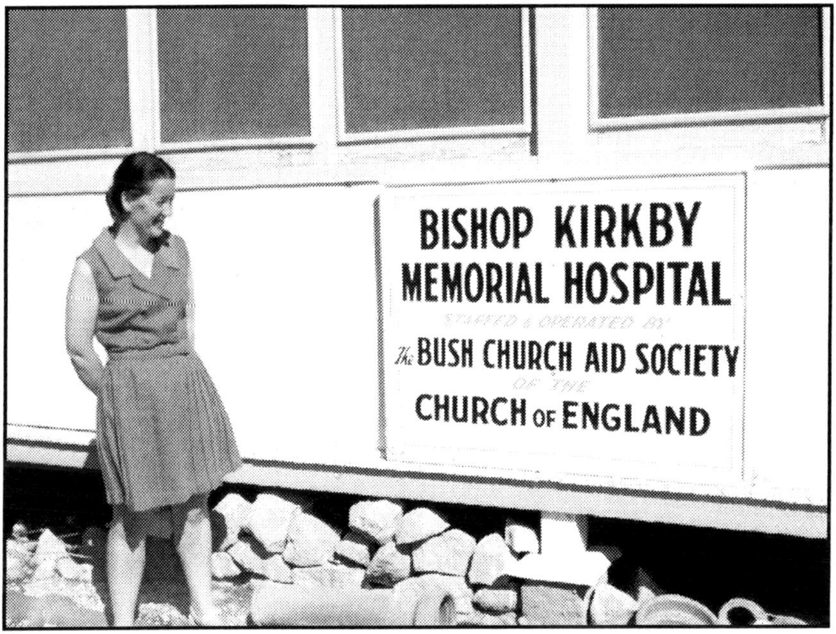

Ruth beside the Cook Hospital sign

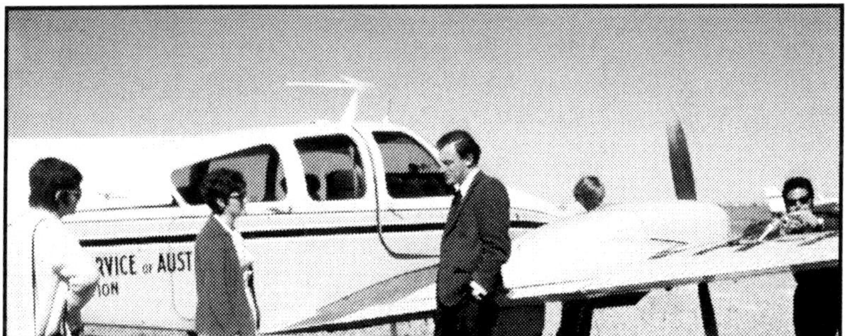

Flying Doctor, Nurse, and plane at Cook

CHAPTER 18 THE FINAL TRIUMPH

Sitting in the kitchen talking to Carol again was like heaven. All the stress dissipated and I felt the warmth of the sunny blue sky outside just by looking out the window at it. Seeing Barry and Jenny again, renewing an old friendship with Val from Melbourne, and meeting Pat for the first time—nothing was traumatic—just pure joy. The work which I thought would be so difficult was an enjoyable challenge. I had come through the cold valley of Christian trial, and landed up on the top of a beautiful mountain of God's blessing. In the middle of a most inhospitable desert, I'd found some of the flowers anyway.

The next day I started to renew my acquaintance with the Coober Pedy routine. The extra busyness of this place led to a totally different emphasis from the other two B.C.A. hospitals. I suddenly knew I had learnt enough to succeed.

There were four of us here now, a great improvement since the days of Anne and Shirley's lonely battles. It was run as one doing outpatients, one inpatients and helping the other with the outpatients, one in charge of the domestic scene, and the fourth one off duty. We also had some help here with the cleaning and hospital washing by employing local workers, but all the cooking was done by us. My cooking was still not brilliant, but I managed, and the medical work was intriguing.

Midwifery being my favourite as by now you all know well, I couldn't resist. When I heard there was a mid in, it took me all my time to stay out of it, even when I was on my days off. I heard she was in—the French lady in labour early, with her first babe. We never delivered first babies in the outback as these were not proven successes because of no previous obstetric history, so this lady had been booked to go to Port Augusta a month before her due date. She was just about to embark on that journey, when the labour started, and she presented at Coober Pedy Hospital. "I will not interfere unless asked" I said to myself, but God already knew how much I wanted to be involved, as indeed He also would have known just what He was going to give me the strength and ability to achieve.

The plane was sent for and when it arrived she was in such good labour that the plane turned back. Much more dangerous to deliver mid air it was decided. Not long after, the labour became obstructed, and we had a dilemma on our hands. "Would you be able to do a forceps Audrey?" Carol asked. Would I? Just give me the chance. I had assisted with many, and at that time knew the procedure off by heart. Wade, the flying doctor, spoke to me by phone. " Whatever you do don't pull hard," he said, but he gave me permission to go ahead.

The others treated me like the visiting obstetrician, and gowned and gloved I assessed the situation. The membranes were ruptured, the patient in labour, the bladder and bowel empty, the cervix fully dilated, the foetal heart was present but dropping, and there was no time to lose. We explained to this lady that this was not usually our job, but in her case there was no other safe option. She gave her consent. I checked the position of the presenting part. Thank God it was a head, but what way was it lying? I had examined many women in labour but never with the head down so low. The feeling was quite foreign to my fingers as I searched for some recognisable marker. Suddenly I had it—a tiny ear on the upper side, to the patient's right. I now knew that this baby was in the best position possible for a successful forceps delivery.

I cut the episiotomy as I had done so many times as a Staff Midwife at the Royal Women's Hospital in Melbourne. The forceps lubricated, I gently inserted them one at a time, as I had seen done so often before, but they didn't fit together and I knew they must before I could proceed. So, as I had also seen even the most accomplished practitioners do in days gone by, I took them off and tried again. This time a perfect fit, and I knew I was ready. The next contraction came. I remembered Wade's words so I didn't pull, and nothing happened. Due to the baby's slowing heart rate, I also knew that the next contraction had to be it, so when it came I pulled with all my might, successfully extracting quite a blue little babe. A quick assessment of this baby told me she would never breathe without some kind of intervention. This situation was also not unfamiliar to me, and I was comforted by the words of a wonderful lecturer, Doctor Glynn White, whom I had had while doing Infant Welfare. "All you need is oxygen and suction, all you need is oxygen and suction…" he had said. I complied, and with the help of frog breathing, another RWH trick, I resuscitated this babe to a pink screaming bundle and turned to deliver the afterbirth and sew up the episiotomy. The whole process was a tremendous blessing, not the least of it being that there was not a single forceps mark on the baby's face. What a miracle.

Through the night I went back to check. "This baby is very yellow," said Val, looking at me with a questioning concern. Again that lecturer's voice with the broad Australian accent rang in my ears. "Jaundice in the first eight hours is a danger sign." Transferred immediately to Adelaide, the child needed three exchange transfusions for an ABO blood incompatibility, a condition about which we could not have known or been able to prevent. Thanks to, I believe, divine providence, we had delivered this baby safely and managed a serious complication. Seen 12 months later was a healthy little girl, successfully reaching all her milestones. What a privilege to do this task and what a God who enabled and kept this situation safe.

But not only was the obstetric side of things exciting. One never knew day or night what might come through the front door of this bush town hospital. Carol was in charge, and was certainly a very efficient and creative boss. It can't have been easy to co-ordinate such a changing and potentially critical scene, and I admired her for the way she did it.

The phone rang and a panic-stricken voice communicated the latest crisis. A miner had fallen down an eighty-foot drillhole and would need a shot of painkiller before being winched to the top. Carol looked across at me. Would I go down a hole that deep via a narrow dirt opening in the ground not much wider than myself? "Yes" I said. "I'll go." I collected the analgesia and a syringe, changed into my jeans, and went with the ambulance crew out to the eight mile mine. "Don't let your feet hit the sides too much as you go or the dirt will fall below". The instruction echoed in my head as I perched on the narrow piece of wood which was to lower me down the dim shaft. I clutched firmly at the ropes attached to my unstable seat, dangling my feet as straight as possible as the winch dropped my seat slowly downwards to the injured man waiting below.

He said nothing when I reached him. Pale under facial dirt and sweat, his body crumpled up under him, this man showed the pain and anguish that did not need words to express. I administered the analgesic, spoke encouragingly of the soon to come rescuers, and was raised upwards again the same way I had come. Remaining to watch, I was so impressed with the efficiency and gentleness of the Coober Pedy team. We flew our patient to Port Augusta that night for proper assessment and treatment.

Then there were the friends we made. "This is Sue my wife, my name is Joe, and this is our little boy Hamish." It was one of my weeks in outpatients, diagnosing, treating and prescribing for the endless line of waiting clients. I looked into the face, full of friendly humour and openness. "What can I do for Hamish?" I asked. His attractive mother replied. "I think he may have sore ears." I had found it was best with children to look at everything, but you had to be clever and go from the least to the most traumatic parts of the examination or you would miss out on getting a chance to see the rest. Breathing, chest then ears. Yes,

Mum was right. Treatment for the ear infection organised, and the family about to go, Joe looked back at me and said, "Pop in and visit us sometime."

On my day off I went to the caravan which I knew was their home. But Joe's car was parked beside it and I was still shy. If it had just been Sue at home I would have gone straight up to the door. Why was I such a wimp? About to turn and go I thought of a book I was currently reading. Unfortunately I have lost the book now and cannot remember the title, but I know it was a Christian book which spoke of overcoming one's fears in order to better enjoy God's blessings. I took the advice, went up to the door, and knocked firmly.

Joe opened it, and I went in to make friends with one of the nicest couples I have ever met, and I never forgot afterwards, that if I let fear take over, I will probably be the one to miss out on something good.

Another couple I grew close to was Kerry and Noel. Noel drove trucks to and from Coober Pedy and often Kerry was left alone with her little girl while Noel was away. Regular visits to Kerry cemented our friendship which continued right on after my B.C.A. years and through the trauma of Noel's death on the highway one dark day. Kerry had known Noel since they were small children, when romantically he used to carry her books home from school. Kerry was a beautiful girl and their love was one of the truest I have ever seen.

Sitting in their dugout kitchen Noel would tell me how they dug out another room by just extending the hole inwards. "Also hoping to find some opal in the walls Audrey and give up the trucks". If only he had.

It was Doctors day again, but here, as it was weekly, the same fuss was not made. The same Doctor and one of the same set of pilots as visited Cook and Tarcoola, came here too, often now accompanied by a nurse. "Do you think there is a romance going on here?" Carol whispered to me one day about one of the flying doctor pilots and one of the flying doctor nurses. "Looks like it" I whispered back. "Better keep an eye on this"! Sure enough some months later an engagement was announced and our secret thoughts were vindicated. The outback and a lot of its uniqueness was certainly romantic enough, and this was the icing on the cake.

I had hated this place the first time, and now I loved it. The old antagonism of Laverton seemed such a long way in the past. The social life of Coober Pedy, plus the spiritual fellowship was very uplifting. However I was still battling with the old compulsive eating urges, and was happy to find that Pat and Val had decided to go on the weight-watchers diet. "I'll be in that too" I chimed in, much to Carol's disgust, who was the thin one and was naturally fearful of being put on a diet too. We honestly did try to feed her properly, and those of us who needed to all lost quite a lot of weight, so we hoped it was all in a good cause. I never did conquer the eating problem properly though, until some five or so years later, when I got the whole thing together and stayed thin for the rest of time. But that is another story. Nevertheless I did feel that even then God was trying to help me, because one evening I desperately wanted to go and eat some bread even though I knew I didn't really need it. I prayed, "Please stop me", and went to the bread bin only to find that the bread in it was mouldy! I laughed and went on with my work without over indulging at that time anyway.

Carol's voice interrupted my thoughts. "There is a very ill man at Arkaroola who needs to be picked up and flown to Port Augusta," she said. We had the doctor with us again, but no nurse was on board this time so I was to go. If it hadn't been such a sad trip I would have loved another plane ride. Arkaroola is a beautiful resort in the heart of South Australia's Flinders Ranges. As Peter my favourite pilot propelled the tiny aircraft over the treetops, his red hair shining in the sunlight, I thought again of the beauty of God's creation as I had so many times during my B.C.A. adventures. But what would await us on the ground?

The gentleman concerned was a Doctor holidaying, when he

had developed an enlarging lump in his abdomen and an increasing feeling of unwellness. He knew what was wrong and had asked for an evacuation. We took on board a charming man with no palpable pulse or recordable blood pressure. Up in the air he was quite conscious due to the lower pressure in the aircraft. I tried to access a vein to no avail. This lovely man had a huge aortic aneurysm which was stealing all his blood away from the vital organs. I knew he didn't have long to live. We touched down at Port Augusta where an ambulance was waiting to take him the rest of the way to Adelaide. I heard later that he had died on the trip.

The next day Carol held a meeting. "We're going to be handed over to the Government," she said. "B.C.A. up to its old tricks" quipped Pat. "What will that mean to us," said Val. "Shiftwork" we all moaned.

I got up at 6 AM, made my coffee, and had my quiet time as always. Luckily I had managed to maintain this over all these months, even when things were tough. Dressing carefully into my white nurse's uniform, I felt special this morning. Today I was to work the first shift of the Coober Pedy Public Hospital.

The work didn't change of course except that we employed a cook for lunch, so no longer did we have to do the domestic chores except to get breakfast in the am and the evening meal while on the appropriate shift. This was sometimes a bit of a juggle because you could be in the middle of making toast when someone with burns arrived on the doorstep. "Just a matter of organisation" said Carol sternly. I was so fed up with her but I found out she was right. "And by the way" she added, "Who fed that kitten?" "I fed it and I'll deal with it" I answered her sharply.

What was I going to do? This beautiful little fluffy thing had appeared at the back door, and Jenny had said it had been around for a few days. I knew it probably didn't have a home any more, and I also knew that after the last hospital cat who slept on the babies clean cots whenever it could sneak in, Carol had absolutely outlawed cats. She herself still had her small dog called Mokey, but then dogs could be trained to stay in certain areas and I had to admit Mokey was well-trained.

My mother had always looked after all the stray animals who turned up at our country vicarage homes, and it had been quite a daunting experience. Dad, a most gentle man who would not have willingly hurt a fly and was as much an animal lover as any of us, was recurrently given the job of culling the numbers. This he did by a special arrangement with the local Chemist who supplied him with a small bottle of Chloroform for which he had to sign the book. I didn't have any Chloroform, but I had seen a bottle of Ether in the clinic cupboard. Now all I needed was an airtight tin and the emotional strength to do this terrible thing. I did it as soon as possible, but I was very saddened to see that pretty little kitten go. Barry came over to help me dig the hole. Coober Pedy soil was not exactly easily diggable. I cried.

Unfortunately having dealt with this so efficiently I was shortly after co-opted again with the appearance of a large wild stray cat. This was more complicated as this cat needed to be locked in the garage without food until hungry and then fed with Valium-laced cat food. While he was sleeping this off I was just able to catch and entomb this poor creature also, though he was still quite strong as I put him in the tin with the ether. It was Doctors day again and Pilot Peter was out nosing around. "How can you be so cruel?" he threw at me accusingly. "Can you make any better suggestions?" I flung at him, and without answering he went back inside. I was glad that I didn't ever have to do this again.

As mentioned before on my first trip to Coober Pedy, the nurses were also the local vets, so we all had to attain a licence in immunisation of animals. Fortunately, as this was quite a regular duty, it was a much pleasanter task than the aforementioned one.

What I didn't find pleasant was the immunisation clinics for the babies of the town. Boy did I hate those days, and they seemed to come up with alarming regularity. I wasn't against the process in principle, but I vowed then that I would never take another job that required me to jab dear little unsuspecting humans with horrible sharp needles when they least expected it. Somehow I've managed to stick to that vow.

"Got time today for a drive—I want to show you something?" said Carol. I was on a day off and as usual it was beautiful weather, so off we went. "Where are you taking me" I asked, knowing her well enough to realise I probably wasn't going to get a straight answer. "Besides," I said to her, "Where are the Fish and Chips". We seemed to have this rapport that I suppose comes from long term compatible working relationships, where we usually knew the meaning of one another's obtuse remarks without having to explain ourselves. She knew I was referring to those 'salad days' at Cook, when trying to simulate urban normality we used to cook fish and chips in our hospital kitchen, wrap them up in newspaper, drive out of town a few miles and sit in the car in the middle of nowhere and eat them out of the packet! We drove on remembering, past the various mining areas and through the barren landscape, when miraculously the terrain began to change and in the distance was a panorama of rugged bluish-grey hills. In front of this distant scene was an absolute carpet of flowers, purple, white, yellow etc. I knew it had rained recently in one of those rare times, and from the reddish brown earth a natural garden had sprung forth like magic. It was breathtaking. Sometimes the rare rains did too good a job and caused floods, blocking the road from bringing in food supplies, and also either preventing the doctor from coming in, or from going out. Once when this happened, the doctor and pilot were already at the hospital and had to spend a whole extra unplanned week at Coober Pedy playing cards and making a general nuisance of themselves in a playful kind of way. We decided we would try not to let them get in at all in the future if rain was forecast!

I snapped out of my ponderings and asked Carol where we were. "This is called the Breakaways," she said. "Isn't it beautiful"? I had to agree.

***

"Not more midwifery", said Val. She slid up beside me and whispered "I hope we get to do this one together because we can do a Royal Women's Hospital Melbourne delivery." I had to admit that that would appeal to me because different schools did things differently. Certainly having a baby was much the same anywhere, but the smoothness of the operation often depended on the officiating professionals knowing who was going to take care of which part of the proceedings. People from the same hospital always knew their hospital routine exactly, so there was no question about who did what, when and where, and efficiency was enhanced. Val and I had met previously when both working at The Royal Women's Hospital in Melbourne, so we were confident that our individual routines would be perfectly understood by both of us.

Jenny Rainsford was to have her third baby with us, and for such a nice lady to choose to do this, as well as her being our dear friend and Christian colleague, we were looking forward to it. Sure enough Val was on and I was her on call when Jenny's time came, and even if I say so myself Val and I shared a brilliant delivery, her delivering and me assisting, there in that faraway place, for someone special.

The next morning I caught the bus to stay with Sid and Flo Bailey in Port Augusta. Flo had been a B.C.A. outback worker many years prior, but had always maintained contact with the current nurses, and together with her husband Sid, provided a haven in their Port Augusta home for weary workers. Sid was an incorrigible tease, and could never understand how we could go to bed our first night at their place at about 7.30 PM and sleep solidly through the night to about the same hour the next morning. That also puts me in mind of the way we could always achieve the same sound sleeps each time we went overnight on the trans trains. What Sid did not understand was the sort of hours we often worked. It was nothing to be up 24 hours or more at a time, sewing up cut heads, attending to car accidents, delivering babies which any obstetrician will tell you is quite often a nocturnal sport, not to mention looking after inpatients when there was insufficient staff to employ any of us on permanent night shift and probably not enough regular call for it anyway. While Sid teased, Flo just quietly took it all in and supported us through everything. What a wonderful couple they were.

My few days holiday over, I hopped on a half empty bus at midnight for the 12-hour trip back. I grabbed a whole seat to myself and was preparing for another of those long sleeps, when a rotund little man in his ?thirties sat down determinedly beside me. "Blast", I thought to myself. "There is plenty of room on this bus for this man to be sitting on his own, how dare he spoil my chance of another good sleep." It was then that the Lord spoke, so I said to Him, "OK, I'll say Hello and if he continues the conversation I'll talk to him, and if he doesn't I'll have done my bit and be able to go to sleep." "Hello" I said, and from then on ensued a long discourse on all this man's hang-ups about Christianity and his inherited Catholicism. He turned out to be a miner from Andamooka, and in between meaningful discussion, he did keep asking if he could contact me in Coober Pedy some time. I continued to affirm that if he had any further queries he should contact Barry Rainsford our trusty B.C.A. pastor. Finally we arrived at Andamooka, and as he got out he shook my hand warmly, thanking me for all the talks. I never saw him again either. I hope of course that he found what he was looking for in God. Probably won't know this one before eternity comes around.

When I got back it was my birthday the next day. "Be ready," said Pat with a knowing smile. Pat was definitely the caterer amongst us, and the dear thing had invited Sue, Joe and family, Barry, Jenny etc, to a special birthday tea. We held it in the newer area of the hospital living quarters and it was a lovely evening. I still remember it as being one of the nicest birthdays I ever had.

***

I rang the flying doctor again, for the second time in the day. "More dramas?" quipped our pleasant young reliever. "Yes I'm stumped by this one," I said. I have a man in the treatment room whose cut his arm quite deeply, and when I try to sew it up there is a bleeding point which I can't quite see to tie off, and the blood welling up is spoiling my view." "Just put on a blood pressure cuff blown up to a safe level," he replied. You can leave it on for 20 minutes at a time, while you do what is necessary. Simple eh?" Indeed it was and it worked like a charm. So nice to have clever doctors the other end of the phone. Actually he wasn't only clever but also a very nice person. Two of the Flying Doctor service nurses had invited me to a camping trip at Victor Harbour, and he had come with us. We had shared a wonderful weekend, especially when us three girls sleeping in the two man tent woke the first morning to the raucous laughter outside of our male companion. "You look so funny from this angle," he said. Apparently as the three of us had rolled over we had tilted the tent on to its side and were blissfully unaware. "Aren't you lucky you're sleeping in the car?" we said to him. I think he was very well aware of that.

Back on the job I continued to cruise through each day with a feeling of sheer pleasure. The spiritual work was also a joy. Pat came home from church one Sunday reporting that a guy whose arm burns we had dressed for some weeks, was enquiring about me at church. Strange I thought, but I decided to wait and see what happened. Next week I was off on Sunday morning, so I went along to the service as usual, and met up with this same young man afterwards. "I like you immensely" he said, "and I would like to go out with you." Not another Miles experience I thought, but kept my cool. I discovered he had some personal problems and because I felt he would probably be better off fixing himself up first before getting involved with someone else, I suggested he join us for Bible study instead, and he did. One of the other guys at Bible study said to us, that this man was after one of us nurses, but we just kept quiet, and the man became a Christian, and then met someone else in town who was right for him and his new found faith. Before leaving Coober Pedy he came to the hospital to thank me for pointing him in the direction he had taken. I knew then that for the moment I was to continue alone reaching out to others. Probably a single woman was quite effective in Christian outreach to all these men, as long as she managed not to become involved. I found out later that it wasn't my turn to have a permanent special someone for many years to come, but was thrilled to bits that the young man with the burns had found, through our ministry, the pearl of great price.

I mustn't omit for the romantics reading this that I did have one proposal. Dressing a man's wounds one day he brightly asked, "Sister are you married?" to which I replied "No." He promptly followed on with "Will you marry me?" whereupon I laughingly and without any need to think, likewise replied. "No." We both had a chuckle, and he good-naturedly went his way.

***

A new day dawned with the usual blue sky and bright sunshine. It was Coober Pedy race day and I was to sell soft drinks at the hospital charity kiosk. I was looking forward to seeing this Coober Pedy highlight. This was no ordinary event, but a golden opportunity for anyone who wished, to become a jockey for a day. If it hadn't been for the accidents it would have been quite hilarious. Unfortunately in they came by ambulance, one after the other, fractured this, fractured that, so my day at the races became a day back at the hospital, assisting with all the wounded being prepared one after the other for evacuation to Port Augusta. I guessed the locals still thought it was worth it, but I'm not sure that the casualties were too thrilled with the painful outcomes.

At the hospital we prayed together as a group of four nurses every night after dinner. Often I must admit I didn't feel at all like it, but once we got started I always ended up loving it, and finding practical direction for everyday problems. We often had Aboriginals come to the back door asking for money, and I always felt this to be a dilemma. One night we read the Bible passage for the day and it said, 'give to those who ask whatever their need.' Afterwards, as I was on duty, I stayed behind while the others went out. There was a tap at the back door and I went to answer. The Aboriginal standing there asked for money. "How much would you like?" I enquired, wondering what I would do if it were a lot. "$2" he said, "to go to the movies." I thought of the Bible verse and gave him the money.

At the hospital there were naturally some incompatibilities amongst the four of us, but we managed to work along with these without too much disruption. We laughed, we had fellowship, we had fun. The drive-in theatre, the basketball games where we watched John, the schoolie from Cook, do his stuff, the breakaways, the wildflowers, the beautiful warm sun. What an oasis for a weary Christian worker to be allowed, after all the preceding harsh lessons, to be nurtured in this way…if only this could go on for ever. I now felt that I had at last found all the flowers in the desert.

***

Months passed and then the letter came. Mum needed me home to help with a house move which was too difficult for her and Dad to cope with due to failing health.

I didn't want to go home. I know I had signed up for two years only and had so far done nearly three. But why now? It was a blow.

Nevertheless I knew that God must have his reasons, which would probably one day be made known to me, if and when that were ever necessary. Meanwhile, each night of the last week, all my new-found friends took me out for dinner separately. It was very sad.

Almost exactly three years since that first lonely day at Cook, I left Coober Pedy by bus. This time I cried. It was the close of the most fulfilling three years of my life so far, and despite all the early traumas, I wouldn't have missed any of it for the world.

COOBER PEDY, S.A.

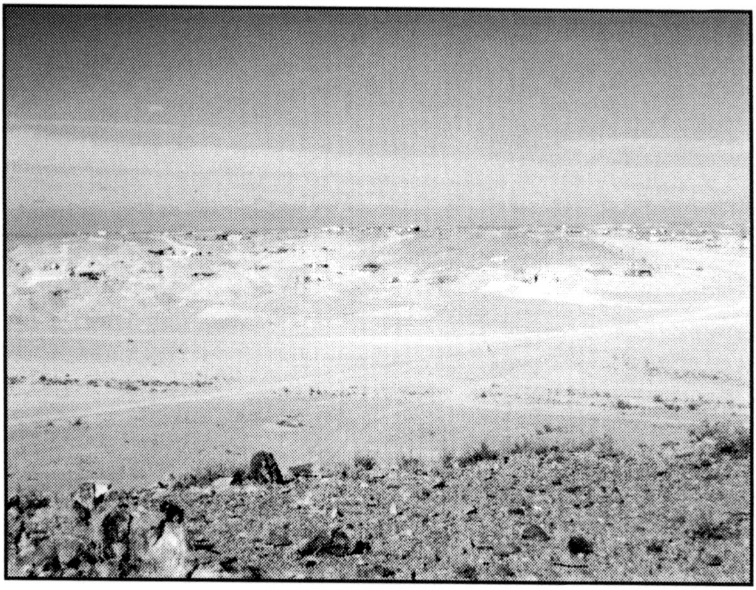

Coober Pedy township, 1973

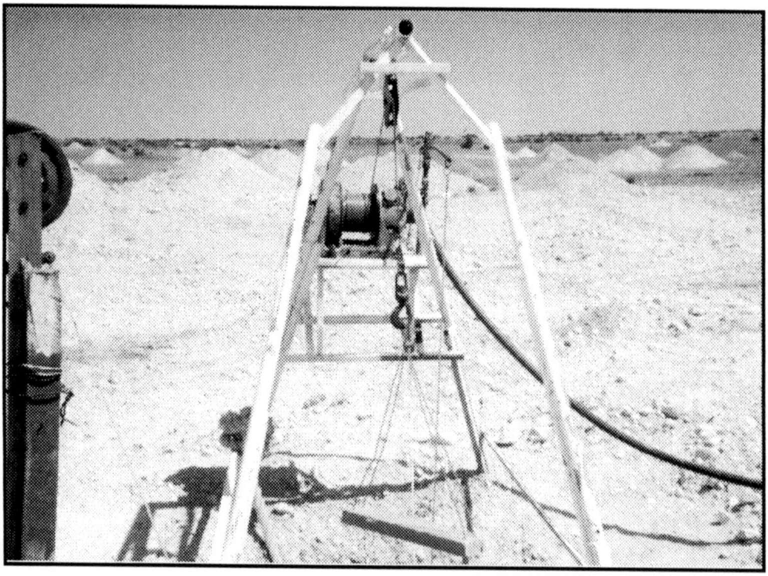

Winch above a drillhole at Coober Pedy

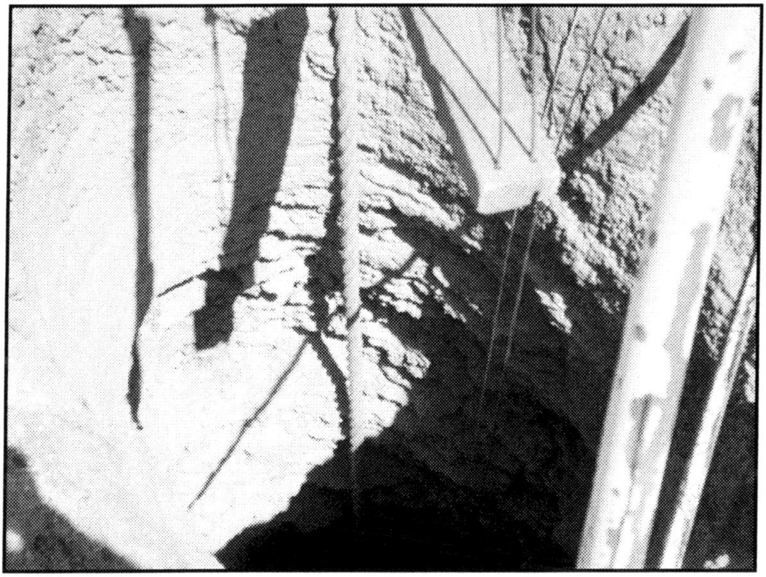

Mining drillhole at Coober Pedy

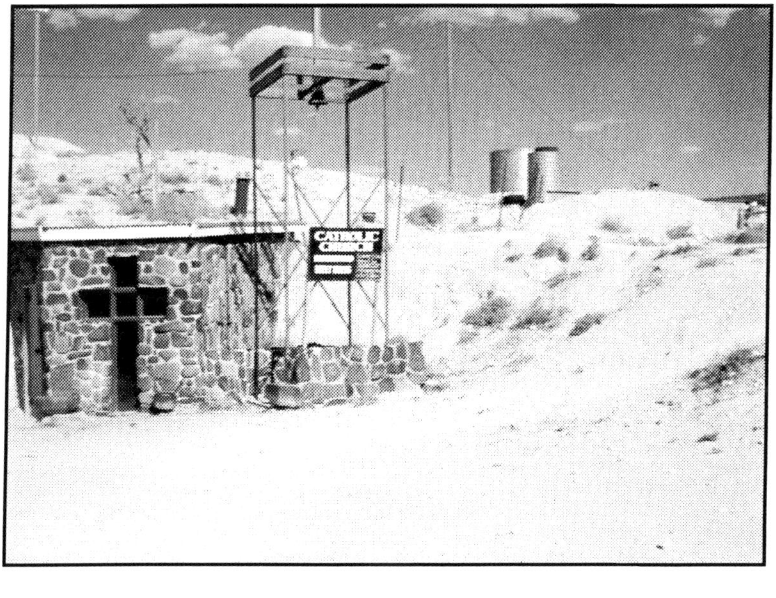

The Roman Catholic dugout Church at Coober Pedy

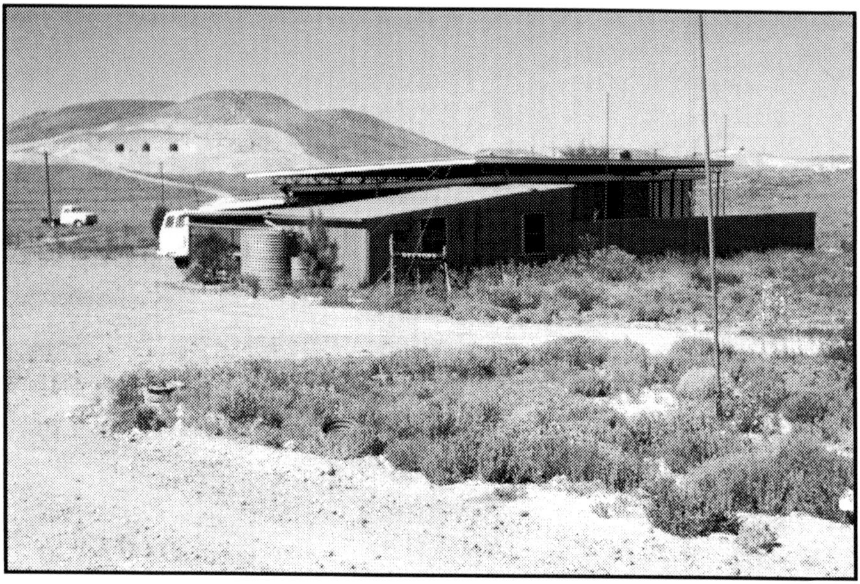

The Rectory at Coober Pedy

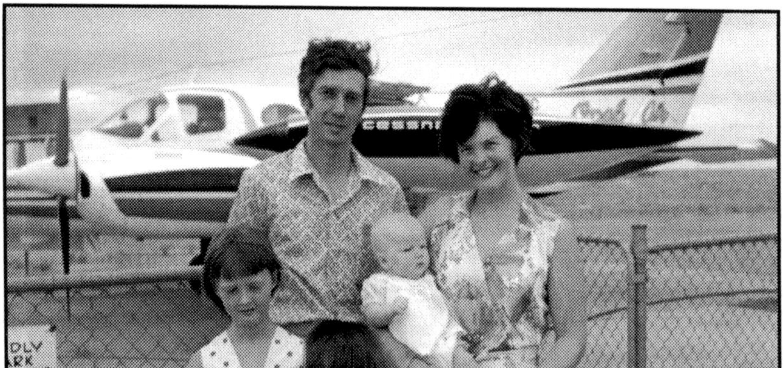

The Rainsfords

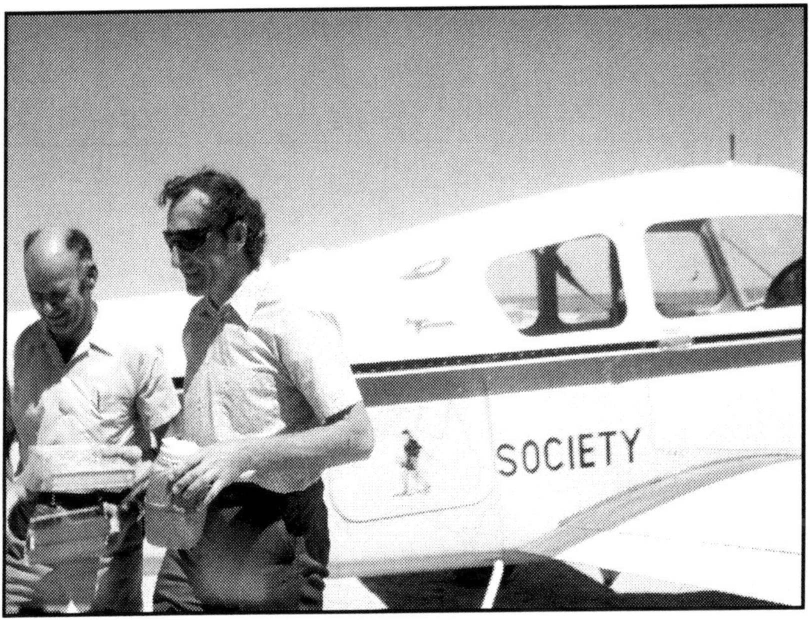

Trevor Booth and Ray Neve with the Bible Society plane

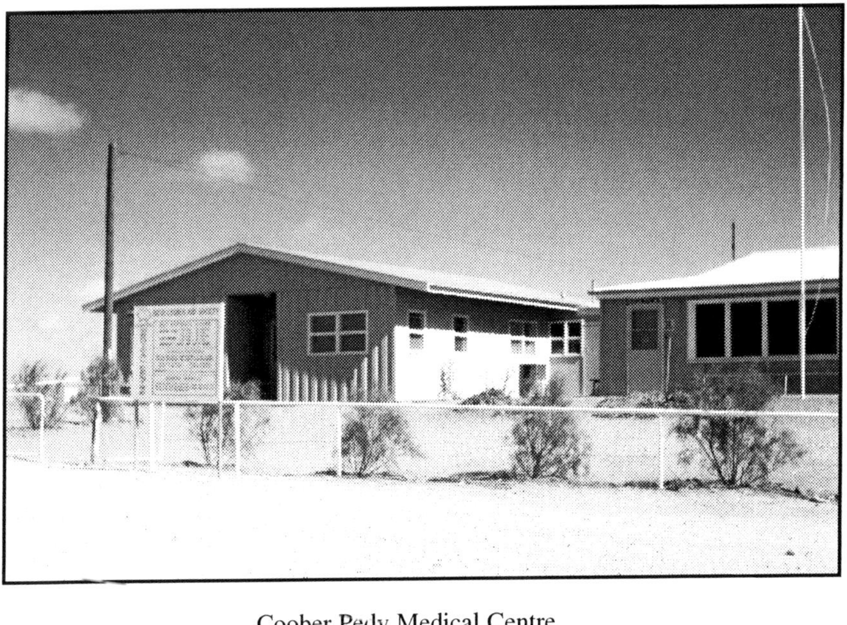

Coober Pedy Medical Centre

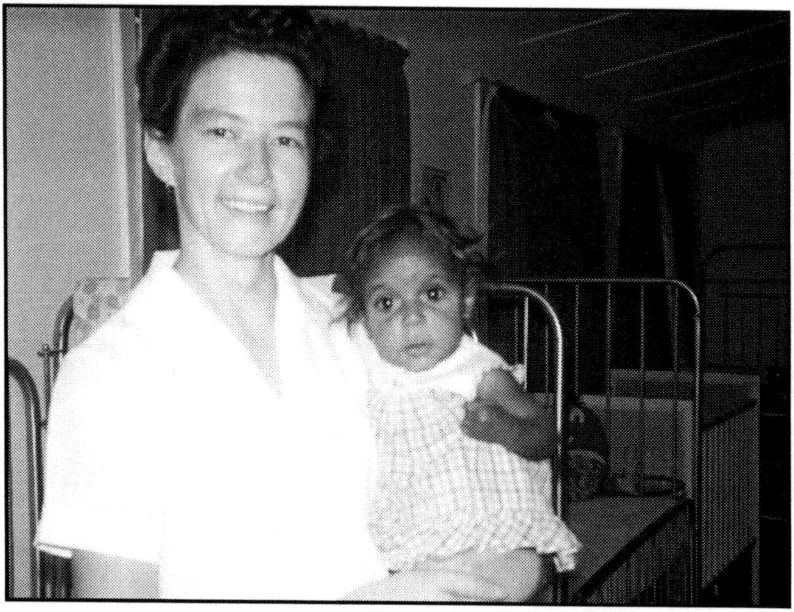

Carol and a patient at Coober Pedy Medical Centre

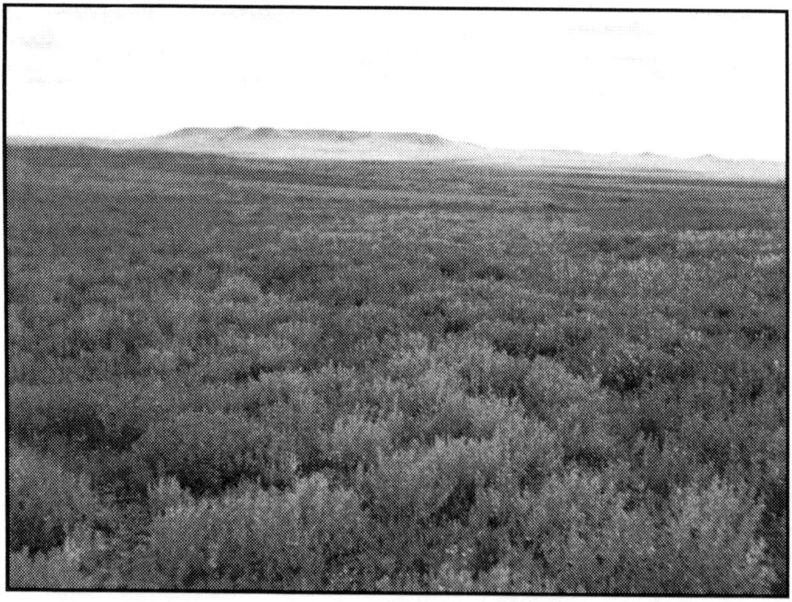

The Breakaways—outside Coober Pedy

EPILOGUE

After returning home to Melbourne, the author spent a year relocating her parents to another place of residence, and assisting them both in their declining health. In 1975, just four months after the move, her father suffered a massive stroke which rendered him hospital-bound until his death in 1976.

Working with the local church, and still not finding a partner of God's choice, Audrey continued to develop her nursing career by undertaking a post graduate diploma at the College of Nursing Australia in 1977, and becoming a Charge Nurse at Cabrini Hospital in 1978. Realising her ailing mother needed her more, she then moved to a home nearby, and continued to assist in that regard, while professionally teaching nurses for a time, and then becoming a Deputy Director of Nursing at Lilydale Hospital, Victoria. While Audrey was still working at Lilydale, her mother became acutely ill and died within 24 hours.

Feeling she had now completed her God-given responsibility to both her parents, Audrey finally married, and now lives in an outer Melbourne suburb with her husband and stepson. Her faith is still the major influence of her life, and despite continually being confronted with situations which seem to test her beliefs, and attempt to undermine her witness, she still believes in and strives to be true to the Christian Way, discovered on that night so many years ago in Sydney, when she gave herself to Jesus in the words of John Stott's Prayer.

PRESENT STATUS LATE 1990s

LAVERTON W.A.

Laverton is now a gold mining town again, as well as nickel. The last population count was 2069, both Aboriginals and white Australians living and working side by side.

Relations between white and black are marred by the usual attitude problem seen in other areas, but this can be between blacks and blacks as much as blacks and whites. Much work is being done on this social integration problem with employment and training programs open to everyone. These are both Government funded and mining company subsidised, and it is felt that real progress has been made. There are pockets of Aboriginal housing areas, but they also live alongside white communities in some parts.

Western Mining redesigned the whole town in 1975, and now there is a church with three services a week and a resident minister. Attendance is thought to be much the same as in other parts of Australia and the attitude found in the 70s towards Christians has largely disappeared.

COOK S.A.

The Bishop Kirkby Memorial Hospital, and indeed the whole town of Cook, is now a ghost town. Due to privatisation of the railways, and the installation of new types of railway tracks which no longer require continual maintenance, there is no need for resident railway workers to be out there. One caretaker family remains to show people from the trains around the town. It is sad to think that Cook as we knew and loved it will never be the same again.

COOBER PEDY S.A.

Coober Pedy is still one of Australia's premiere opal mining towns. Fortunes wax and wane as economies boom and bust. The population fluctuates accordingly.

Coober Pedy's Aboriginal community is still struggling with the traumas of trying to integrate into white society having virtually lost the value of their own culture. Most Aboriginals live on the reserve opposite the hospital and alcohol, still a problem, is now compounded by petrol sniffing, some drug abuse, and gambling.

The newer hospital is still government owned and operated. There are two resident Doctors in the town so the Flying Doctor Service is only used for evacuations.

The church presence continues to thrive. B.C.A. still provides a resident Anglican minister, and Coober Pedy Christians still share the message of Christ when and where possible.

IMPORTANT INFORMATION

CHRISTIAN CONVERSION is a wonderful thing but the means varies greatly from one individual to another. It is based on the premise that the Bible is the inspired word of God, God made us to be His friends, we disobeyed His plan, so He sent His Son Jesus to die so that we could be forgiven and live, and His Holy Spirit can live in us so we may keep in touch with God's will, receiving spiritual gifts and guidance for our daily lives. The simplest way to adopt this lifestyle is to recognise one's need, admit it to God, and ask Jesus to take over from then on. A prayer which could be said may go something like this.

"Heavenly Father God, I believe You are the creator of the universe and all who live in it including me. I believe that You sent Your Son Jesus to die so that I might have everlasting life and peace amid this world's difficulties. I pray now that You will forgive me all my past sins, and send Your Holy Spirit into my life so I can from now on live for You instead of for myself, and from then on know your love and peace in my life, and spend each day serving you, until death reunites me with all those who know and love you.

Through Jesus Name Amen.

You may not feel immediately different but instead find yourself growing in the faith, or you may suddenly find you have a new love for your fellow man, a new feeling of improved self-esteem, and a new plan for living. Try to align yourself now with other Christians, commence a daily routine of prayer and Bible reading, and seek God's will for your life, and you will know a lasting fulfilment that the luxuries of this world can never give.

Best Wishes in Jesus Name.
Audrey Aspeling.

Institutions which may help you include the following:

Scripture Union
The Bible Society
Evangelical Churches in your area
Any Christians you know
Christian booksellers in your neighbourhood
Christian Television e.g. early AM Saturdays and Sundays in Australia, and other countries as scheduled.

THE WHY HOW AND WHERE

TO CONTACT B.C.A.

WHY You may wish to know more about B.C.A. today
You may wish to support the work
You may wish to buy something from them

YOU MAY EVEN WANT TO WORK FOR THEM!

HOW WRITE PHONE FAX OR EMAIL TO:

WHERE B.C.A. NATIONAL OFFICE SYDNEY NSW
Address: Level 7/37 York Street
Sydney NSW 2000
Phone: (02) 9262 5017
Fax: (02) 9262 5020
Email: bcafed@ozemail.com.au

B.C.A. OFFICE MELBOURNE VICTORIA
Address: 1 Burgundy Street
Heidelberg Vic 3084
Phone: (03) 9457 7556
Fax: (03) 9457 7610
Email: bcavic@ozemail.com.au

AUDREY'S SPEECH FOR THE BOOK LAUNCH

SATURDAY 21ST OCTOBER 2000

Firstly I would like to welcome everyone here today, and thank you all for taking the time to join in what to me is a very special and long-awaited occasion. I look around at the familiar faces, some from so many years back I'm not going to be specific, others from very recent times, and just about every stage in between. The whole thing is completely overwhelming.

When I thought about writing this book some ten years back, I had no idea what I was letting myself in for. I can understand now why people can write books about writing books! The ramifications of this adventure are endless.

It may be interesting to note that the book, started nine years ago now, might never have been completed if I had not broken my foot the first time, and might never have reached the stage of publication if I hadn't broken my other foot in the second instance. I now totally believe that God works in very mysterious ways!

There are many people here today who are either in the book, worked out there in the middle of nowhere back in the 1970s, or who supported me and the others from afar, while they held the fort at home. Your presence is so precious. I had no idea when I started all this that it would have such far-reaching and deeply fulfilling potential.

That doesn't mean however, that this has all been easy.

Christian or no Christian, I know that in the middle of the night or early hours of the morning, when I was trying to complete a chapter, or meet some other kind of writing deadline, and the computer decided to do something most peculiar which I'm sure I had nothing whatsoever to do with, that many a time I had an almost overwhelming urge to talk most rudely to it, or walk out into my back yard and drop it unceremoniously into the fishpond. Praying definitely did help, but unfortunately it was not always my first response.

I have written this book for many reasons. Among them was the urge to tell a story which I felt was both unique and romantic, while at the same time scary and depressing. Many times as I wrote, I cried. Someone suggested without my telling her, that the experience of writing about this must have been cathartic, and I was astonished by her insight.

I also felt other people would be interested in what I had found to be a fascinating lifestyle, and I only hope I have captured it all adequately enough for people to understand at least some of the magic.

Finally I have written it unashamedly to share my faith. I not only do this because Jesus told us to, but also because after thirty-two years since my conversion experience in Sydney, I am still as excited about it as I was the first day I found it. For sure I certainly have my moments, and getting this book to the final stage of publication has brought some of the toughest times with it, not to mention the situations I and others shared in the bush which were often tougher than anything else life has thrown at us. I simply wanted an opportunity to tell some of my story, in the hope that others may enjoy the fruits of God's spirit in their lives too. My hope also is that all who read the book, will find something of value in it for them.

Thank you all once again for coming along.

THERE ARE FLOWERS IN THE DESERT

By
AUDREY ASPELING

A True story of Nursing in the Australian outback

In her book Audrey shares her fears, failures, and God-given successes as a Nurse in the Australian Outback for three years with the Bush Church Aid Society in the early 1970s

$20.00 per copy, plus $5.00 postage

ORDER FORM

Name: ....

Address:..

Phone: ....

No. of Books required: ......Cost: ....

Postage: $ ....   Total Cost : $ ....

Method of Payment:

Cheque/Money Order made payable to Audrey Aspeling

Send orders to: Mrs Audrey Aspeling
23 Dublin Road
Ringwood East Vic 3135
Australia